# PRACTICAL AROMATHERAPY FOR EVERYDAY LIVING

*A Comprehensive Guide to Essential Oils and Their Applications for a Balanced Lifestyle*

Michael Hulbert

Special Thanks to the folks at Creation Farm for all their help in generously providing materials for testing and illustration etc. on this project.
You can find more about this company and the items pictured throughout the book at www.creationpharm.biz or search for Creation Farm, or Creation Pharm on Amazon, eBay, Walmart, Etsy, Facebook, or Google.

# Contents

Foreword ............................................................................................. 11

Introduction ........................................................................................ 13

## Chapter One The Basics of Essential Oils .................................. 15
What Are Essential Oils of Plants? ........................................................ 15
How Essential Oils Are Extracted ......................................................... 15
The Quality and Strengths of Essential Oils .......................................... 17
Carrier Oils: Complementing Your Essential Oils ................................. 18

## Chapter Two Safety and Precautions ........................................ 19
General Guidelines for Essential Oil Use ............................................... 19
Dilution and Application Methods ........................................................ 20
Essential Oils to Avoid or Use with Caution .......................................... 20
Safe Use of Essential Oils for Children, Pregnant, Nursing Women, and Elderly ..... 20

## Chapter Three Essential Oils for Aromatherapy ...................... 22
Top Essential Oils for Everyday Use: Benefits, Applications, and Blending Techniques ........................................................................................ 22
Lavender Essential Oil ......................................................................... 23
Peppermint Essential Oil ..................................................................... 25
Eucalyptus Essential Oil ...................................................................... 27
Tea Tree Essential Oil .......................................................................... 29
Lemon Essential Oil ............................................................................. 31
Frankincense Essential Oil ................................................................... 34
Rosemary Essential Oil ........................................................................ 36
Roman Chamomile Essential Oil .......................................................... 38
Sweet Orange Essential Oil .................................................................. 40
Ylang-Ylang Essential Oil ..................................................................... 42

## Chapter Four Herbs and Plants for Essential Oil Production .................................................................. 45

A Comprehensive List of Aromatic Plants and Their Properties ............................... 45
Cultivation and Harvesting Practices ................................................................. 47
Sustainability and Ethical Sourcing of Essential Oils ........................................... 48

## Chapter Five Methods of Aromatherapy ..................................... 49

Inhalation: Diffusers, Steam Inhalation, and Sprays ............................................ 49
Topical Applications: Massage, Compresses, and Baths ...................................... 50
Internal Use: Safety and Guidelines ................................................................... 50

## Chapter Six Aromatherapy for Physical Well-being ............... 51

Pain Relief and Inflammation ............................................................................ 51
Immune Support and Fighting Infections .......................................................... 52
Respiratory Health ............................................................................................ 53
Skin and Hair Care ............................................................................................ 54
Digestive Health ................................................................................................ 55

## Chapter Seven Aromatherapy for Emotional and Mental Balance .............................................................................. 59

Stress and Anxiety Relief ................................................................................... 59
Mood Enhancement and Emotional Support ..................................................... 60
Sleep and Relaxation ........................................................................................ 61
Focus and Mental Clarity .................................................................................. 63
Personal Growth and Self-care ......................................................................... 64
Creating Personalized Essential Oil Blends ....................................................... 65

## Chapter Eight Aromatherapy for Everyday Life ....................... 66

Creating a Morning and Evening Routine .......................................................... 66
Aromatherapy in the Workplace ........................................................................ 67
Travel and On-the-Go Applications ................................................................... 68
Packing and Transporting Essential Oils ........................................................... 69
On-the-Go Aromatherapy Applications ............................................................. 69
Aromatherapy for Special Occasions ................................................................ 70

# Chapter Nine Aromatherapy for Home and Environment..... 73
Natural Cleaning Solutions ......................................................................................... 73
Creating a Relaxing and Inviting Atmosphere ........................................................ 76
Diffusing Essential Oils................................................................................................ 76
Room Sprays ................................................................................................................. 77

# Chapter Ten DIY Aromatherapy Recipes and Projects............ 81
Personal Care Products............................................................................................... 81

# Chapter Eleven Building an Aromatherapy Toolkit................... 92
Essential Oils and Carrier Oils................................................................................... 92
Diffusers and Other Tools .......................................................................................... 92
Storage and Organization .......................................................................................... 92

# Chapter Twelve The Future of Aromatherapy ............................. 92
Emerging Research and Innovations ........................................................................ 92
The Growing Role of Aromatherapy in Integrative Medicine Aromatherapy .......... 92
Aromatherapy and Sustainability.............................................................................. 92

# Conclusion............................................................................................. 92

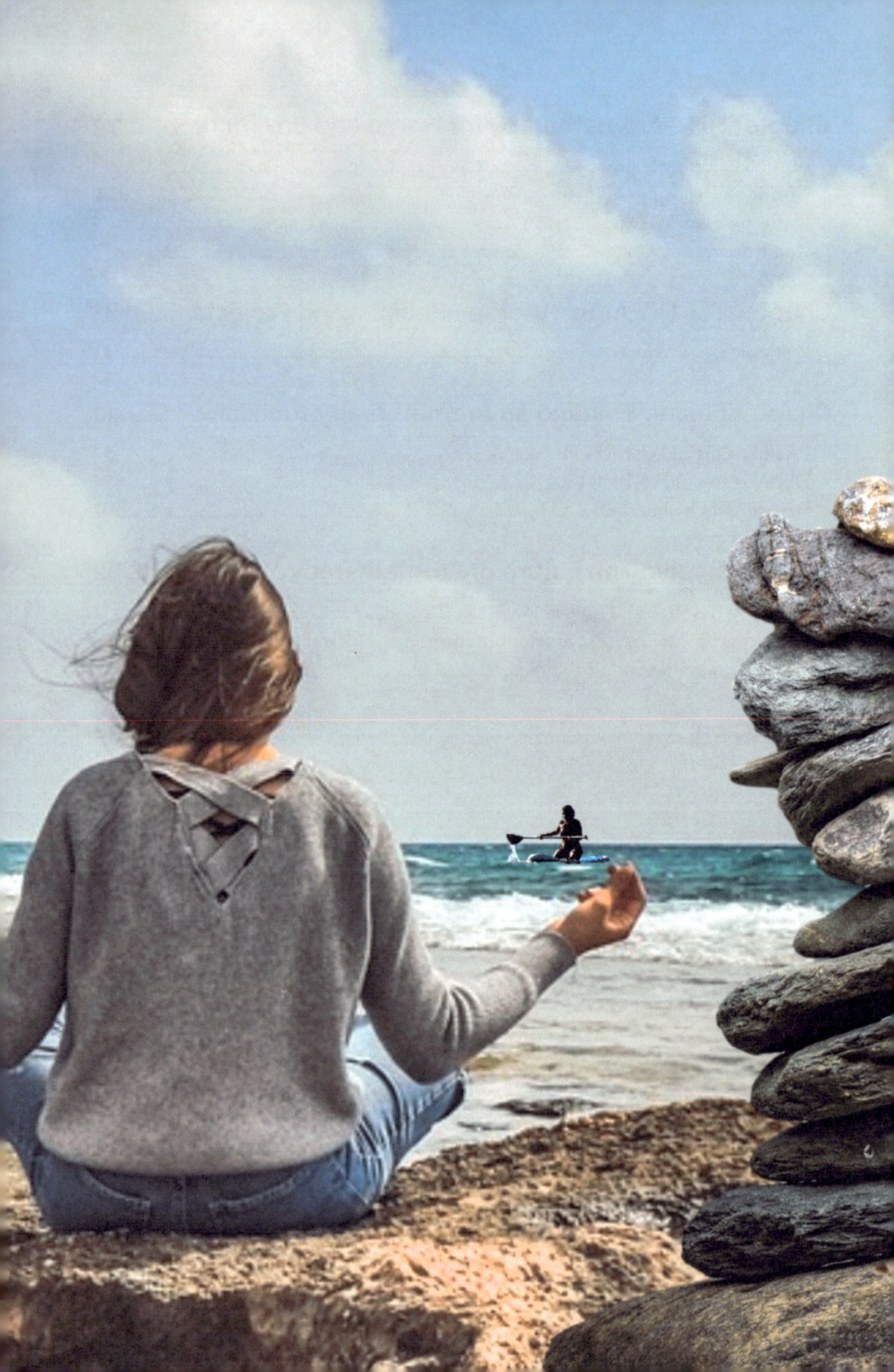

# Foreword

Welcome to Practical Aromatherapy for Everyday Living, a comprehensive guide to essential oils and their applications for a balanced and holistic lifestyle. In the pages of this book, you will discover the amazing power of aromatherapy and how it can enhance your physical, emotional, and mental well-being.

Aromatherapy has been used for thousands of years by cultures all around the world, and it will likely continue to grow as people seek natural and holistic approaches to health and wellness. With the increasing demand for essential oils and aromatherapy products, it's important to have a reliable and informative resource to guide you on your journey.

In this book, you will find everything you need to know regarding essential oils, like distillation, quality and potency factors, and how to use them safely and effectively. You will also discover a wide range of applications for essential oils, from pain relief and skin care to emotional balance and cognitive support.

Whether you're just starting out on your aromatherapy journey or you're a seasoned practitioner, this book has something for everyone. With practical tips, inspiring ideas, and easy-to-follow instructions, you'll be able to incorporate aromatherapy into your daily life with confidence and ease.

So, come join us on this journey into the world of aromatherapy and discover the power of essential oils for your lifestyle. Your mind, body, and spirit will thank you!

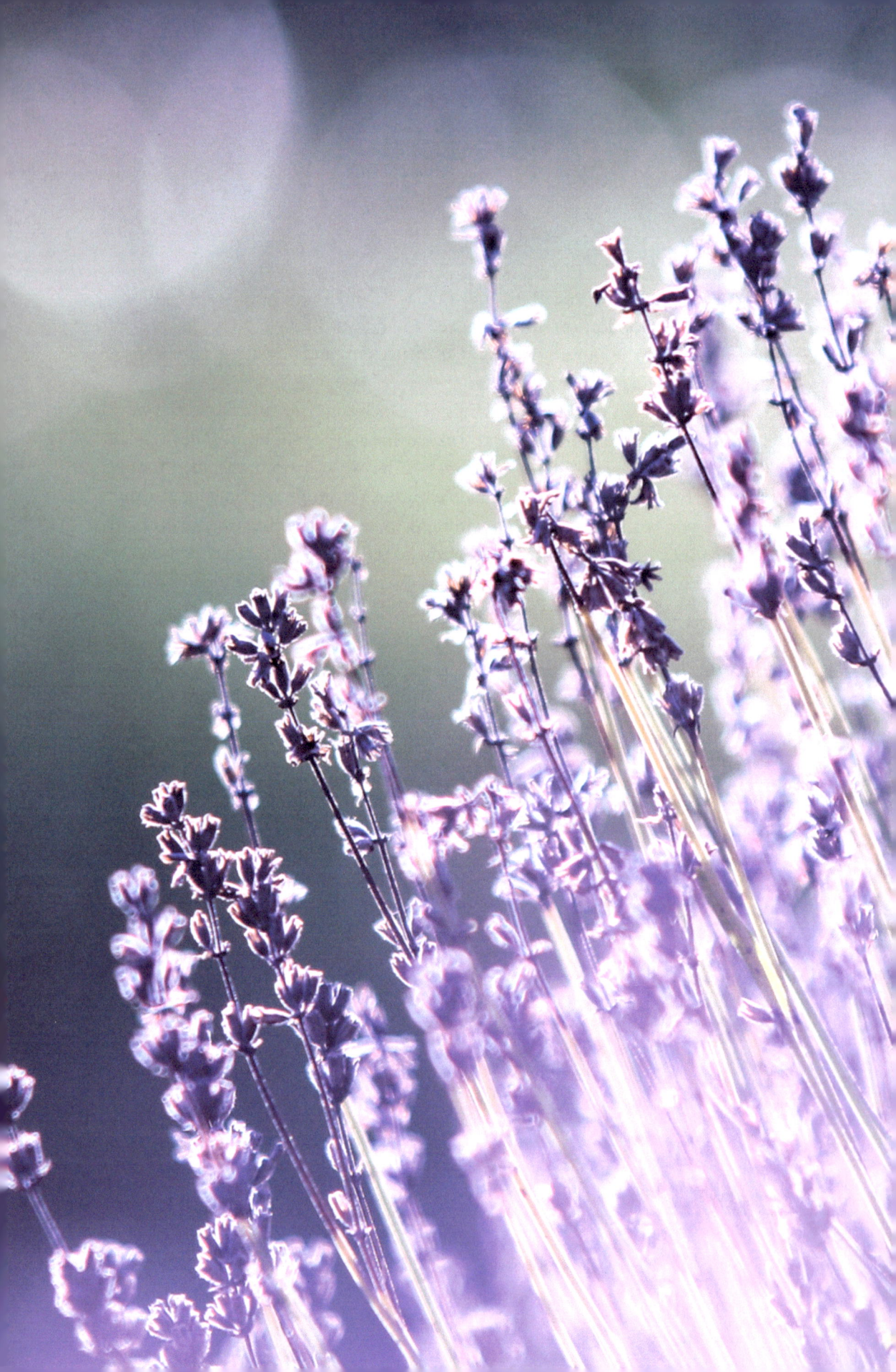

# Introduction

Aromatherapy is an ancient practice with roots that stretch back thousands of years, transcending cultures and civilizations. It is a holistic approach to wellness that seeks to enhance our emotional, mental, and physical well-being through natural plant extracts, specifically essential oils.

In today's fast-paced world, we often search for ways to maintain balance, reduce stress, and promote overall health. Aromatherapy offers a powerful and accessible tool to help us achieve these goals, allowing us to reconnect with nature and harness its healing properties.

The power of aromatherapy lies in its ability to tap into our olfactory system, the part of our brain responsible for the sense of smell. Inhaled essential oil molecules interact with our limbic system, affecting emotions, memory, and hormones. Aromatherapy's unique relationship profoundly impacts well-being, naturally addressing concerns like stress, anxiety, pain, and inflammation.

The book "Practical Aromatherapy for Everyday Living" is a comprehensive guide for anyone looking to incorporate essential oils into their daily routine. It covers the basics of essential oils, their safe and effective use, and explores various oils and herbs used in aromatherapy. The book offers practical tips for everyday life, from personal care to home environment and DIY projects.

You can achieve balance, harmony, and well-being by embracing aromatherapy and using essential oils. This book provides valuable insights and resources to help you create a personalized aromatherapy toolkit and make crucial oils an integral part of your daily routine. Discover the incredible benefits of aromatherapy and transform your life naturally.

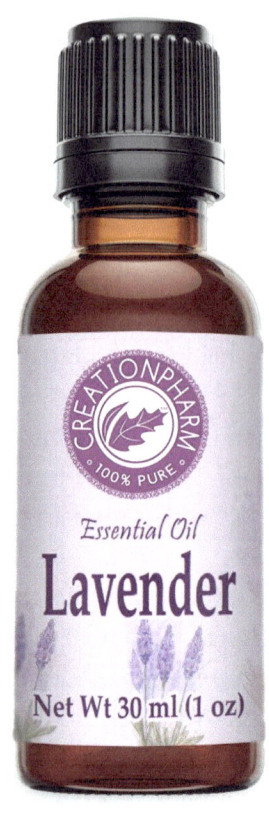
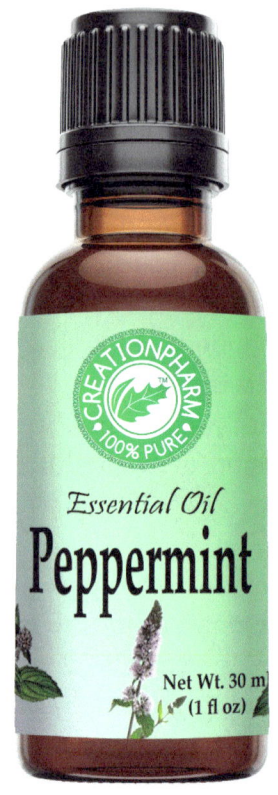
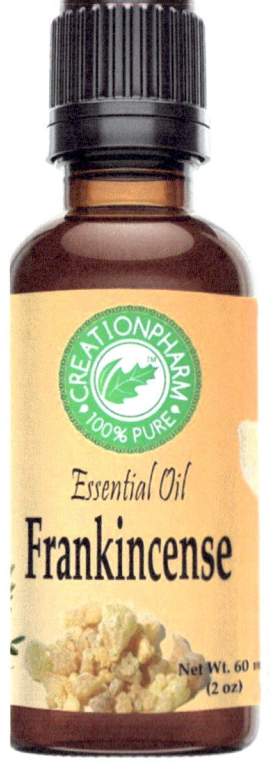
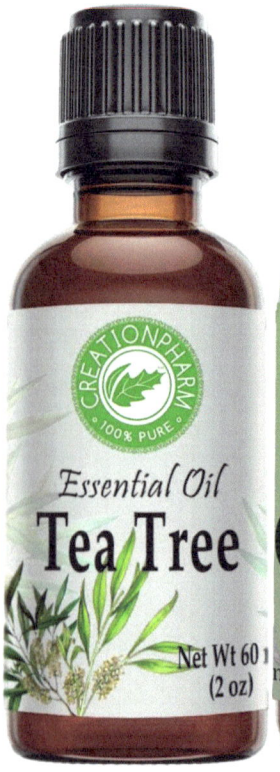
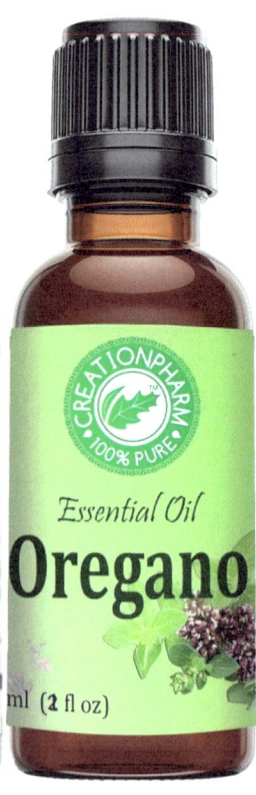

# Chapter One

# The Basics of Essential Oils

Essential oils are at the heart of aromatherapy, providing the powerful scents and therapeutic properties that make this practice so effective. In this section, we will explore the basics of essential oils, including their definition, extraction methods, quality, potency, and the role of carrier oils in aromatherapy.

## What Are Essential Oils of Plants?

Essential oils contain the essence of plants, containing unique aromas and beneficial properties. They've been used in various cultures for thousands of years benefiting from their therapeutic and medicinal properties. With over 90 commonly used oils, each with unique properties, they're extracted through various methods and can be used for personal care, household cleaning, and health and wellness practices. However, essential oils can be harmful if misused, so following safety guidelines and consulting a healthcare professional is important. Discover the fascinating history and uses of essential oils for promoting health and wellness.

## How Essential Oils Are Extracted

There are several methods for extracting essential oils from plants, the most common being steam distillation, cold pressing, and solvent extraction.

**Steam Distillation:** Steam is passed through plant material in this process, causing the essential oil to evaporate. The steam and actual oil vapor are then cooled and condensed into a liquid collected separately from the water. Steam distillation is considered the most efficient, common, and traditional method for extracting essential oils from plant materials.

It involves using steam to separate the volatile oils from the plant material. The botanicals are placed in the distillation chamber, and steam is then injected into the chamber. The steam penetrates the plant material and causes the essential oil to evaporate.

The steam and essential oil vapor mixture is then cooled and condensed in a separate chamber, where it is separated from the water. The essential oil is collected in a container, while the remaining water is discarded or used for other purposes.

Steam distillation is a gentle and efficient process to extract essential oils from delicate plant materials, such as flowers and leaves. It can also remove fats from more challenging materials, such as roots and bark. The resulting essential oil is highly concentrated, with a potent aroma and therapeutic properties.

Some factors that can affect the quality of essential oils produced through steam distillation include the type of plant material used, the quality of the water and steam, and the duration of the distillation process. Properly executed steam distillation results in pure high-quality, essential oils that are used for various therapeutic and aromatherapy purposes.

**Cold Pressing:** Typically used for citrus essential oils, cold pressing involves mechanically pressing the plant material to release the essential oil. No heat is applied during this process, preserving the delicate aromatic compounds.

**Solvent Extraction:** Solvent extraction is often used for delicate flowers that cannot withstand the heat of steam distillation. This method uses a solvent like hexane or ethanol to extract the essential oil so it can be separated from the solvent by evaporation or filtration.

# The Quality and Strengths of Essential Oils

The quality and strengths (potency) of essential oils are crucial factors in their therapeutic effectiveness. Highest quality essential oils are pure, undiluted, without synthetic additives, fillers, or contaminants. Factors that can influence the quality and strength of essential oils include:

- The plant species and variety used for extracting essential oils influence their quality and potency. Some plant species contain a higher concentration of essential oils than others, and even within a single plant species, the variety can affect the composition and potency of the oil. For example, the variety of lavender used for producing essential oil in France has a higher concentration of linalool, responsible for its relaxing properties, compared to the lavender variety grown in Bulgaria.
- Geographic origin and growing conditions can also affect the quality and strength of essential oils. Plants grown in their natural habitat are more likely to produce higher-quality oils than those grown in unfamiliar environments or artificial conditions. The climate, soil, and altitude can also impact the chemical composition of the oils.

- Harvesting and extraction methods also play an important role in the quality and strength of essential oils. Some plant materials must be harvested at specific times to obtain the most potent oils, while others may require special techniques for extracting the oil without compromising its quality. For example, the highest quality rose oil is obtained by handpicking the roses in the early morning before the sun evaporates the delicate oils. Similarly, the best quality citrus oils are obtained through cold-pressing the fruit rind rather than solvent extraction.
- Proper storage and handling are also critical factors in maintaining the quality and potency of essential oils. Heat, light, and air exposure can degrade the quality and strength of oils over time. Essential oils should be stored in dark glass bottles in a cool, dark place away from sunlight and heat sources.
- When it comes to essential oils, quality matters. To ensure you're using effective oils, buy from reputable suppliers who provide information on the oil's origin, extraction method, and testing. Choose certified organic oils to reduce the risk of contamination.

## Carrier Oils: Complementing Your Essential Oils

Carrier oils are a must-have for the safe and effective use of essential oils in aromatherapy. Sweet almond, jojoba, coconut, and grapeseed oil are popular choices, each with unique benefits.

Diluting essential oils with carrier oils is vital to avoid skin irritation, with a general guideline of 2-3% dilution for adults. Choosing high-quality essential oils and appropriate carrier oils is critical to maximizing the benefits of aromatherapy for your well-being.

Chapter Two

# Safety and Precautions

While essential oils offer numerous benefits, using them safely and responsibly is vital to avoid potential risks and complications. This section will discuss general guidelines for important oil use, dilution and application methods, essential oils to be wary of and avoid, or use with caution, and safe service for children, pregnant and nursing women, and the elderly.

## General Guidelines for Essential Oil Use

Essential oils have gained popularity recently for their various health and wellness benefits. However, it's critical to use them safely and responsibly. In this context, general guidelines for essential oil use can help users understand how to use them effectively and avoid potential harm. These guidelines include:
- Always dilute your essential oils with carrier oil before applying them to the skin. Undiluted essential oils can cause skin irritation, sensitization, or burns.
- You can do a patch test by applying a small amount of diluted essential oil to an inconspicuous skin area, such as the inside of your forearm or elbow, and wait 24 hours to check for any negative reactions.
- Keep essential oils out of reach of children and pets.
- Essential oils should not be ingested without the guidance of a qualified healthcare professional or aromatherapist.
- Store essential oils in a cool, dark place away from direct sunlight to maintain their potency and extend their shelf life.

## Dilution and Application Methods

When using essential oils, knowing the proper dilution and application methods is crucial to ensure safe and effective use. Dilution helps to minimize skin irritation and sensitization, while appropriate application methods can maximize the therapeutic benefits of essential oils.

- Essential oils should be diluted in a carrier oil before topical application. A general guideline is a 2-3% dilution for adults ( approximately 12-18 drops of essential oil per ounce of carrier oil).
- For children, elderly individuals, and those with sensitive skin, a lower dilution rate of 0.5-1% (2-4 drops of essential oil per ounce of carrier oil) is recommended.
- Inhalation methods, such as diffusers and steam inhalation, generally do not require dilution. However, it is essential to follow the manufacturer's directions for your diffuser and avoid an overexposure to the aromas.

## Essential Oils to Avoid or Use with Caution

Some essential oils may pose risks or have contraindications for specific individuals or conditions. It is crucial to research each essential oil and consult with a qualified healthcare professional or aromatherapist if you have any concerns.

- Phototoxic essential oils, such as bergamot, lemon, and lime, can cause skin sensitivity when exposed to sunlight. Avoid applying these oils to skin exposed to direct sunlight or UV light within 12-18 hours.
- Some essential oils, like cinnamon, clove, and thyme, can irritate the skin and should be used cautiously at lower dilution rates.
- People with epilepsy, asthma, or other medical conditions should consult a healthcare professional before using essential oils.

## Safe Use of Essential Oils for Children, Pregnant, Nursing Women, and Elderly

Using essential oils safely is crucial, especially for vulnerable populations such as pregnant and nursing women, children, and the elderly. While essential oils can offer many benefits, it's vital to understand how to use them safely and appropriately to avoid potential risks.

- For children under age two it is generally advised to avoid using essential oils. Use a lower dilution rate for older children and opt for gentler essential oils, such as lavender, chamomile, and mandarin.
- Pregnant and nursing women should consult a healthcare professional before using essential oils. Some oils, like clary sage, juniper, and wintergreen, should be avoided during pregnancy.
- Elderly individuals may have more sensitive skin or medical conditions requiring lower dilution rates and extra caution when using essential oils.

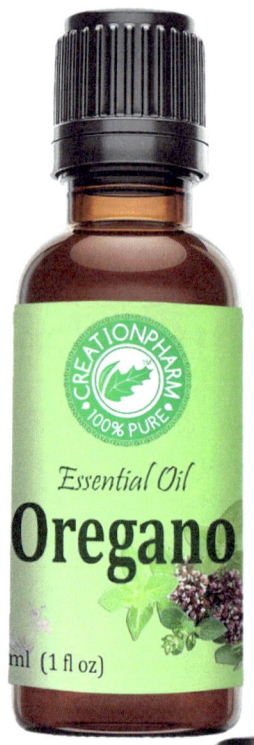
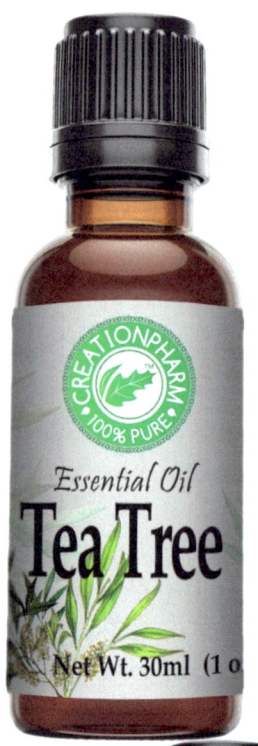
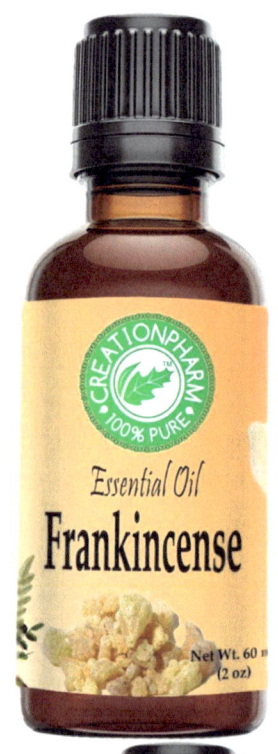
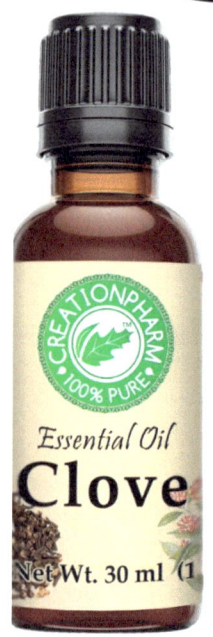
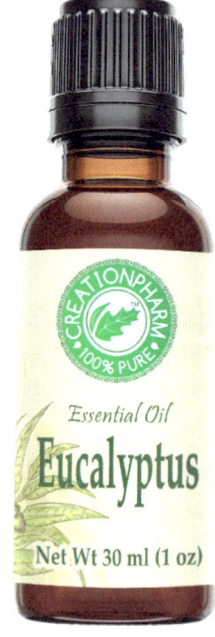
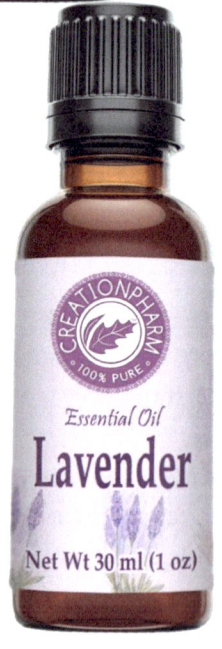
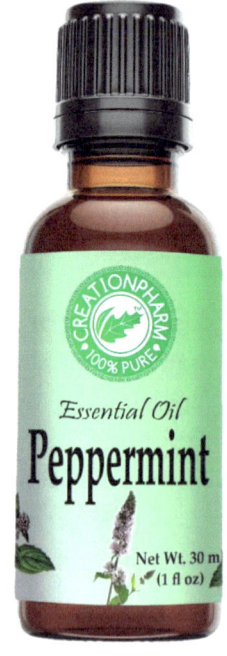

Chapter Three

# Essential Oils for Aromatherapy

Discover the power of aromatherapy and how it can improve your physical, emotional, and mental well-being. Learn about the top essential oils for everyday use, their benefits and applications, and how to blend them for optimal results. With hundreds of essential oils available, this book chapter will guide you on the best choices for safe and easy use. From stress relief to focus and energy, essential oils for everyday use offer a natural and holistic approach to health and wellness.

## Top Essential Oils for Everyday Use: Benefits, Applications, and Blending Techniques

Building a solid foundation for your aromatherapy practice involves selecting the right essential oils for your needs. Some essential oils stand out for their versatility and practicality among the countless options. Below, we have compiled a list of ten top essential oils that offer a wide range of potential applications and benefits. Each essential oil on this list has unique properties that can support physical, emotional, and mental well-being. Here, we highlight some critical properties and uses associated with our top ten essential oils:

# Lavender Essential Oil

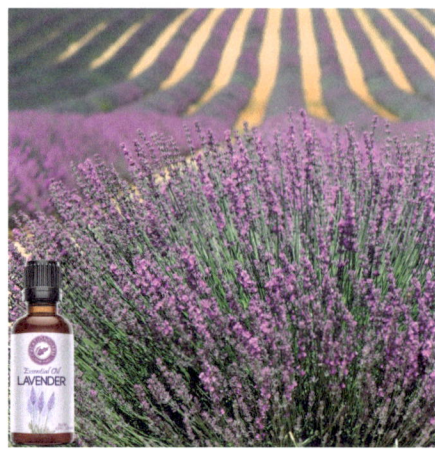

This is derived from the flowers of the Lavandula angustifolia (also known as Lavandula officinalis) plant. This versatile oil is widely used in aromatherapy and skin care for its numerous therapeutic benefits. Lavender's calming, soothing, and healing properties make it popular for various applications.

## Aroma Description

Lavender essential oil has a fresh, floral, herbaceous aroma with a slightly sweet and woody undertone. The scent is often described as clean and calming, evoking tranquility and serenity.

## Countries of Origin

Lavender is primarily cultivated in the Mediterranean region, with the most prominent countries of origin being France, Bulgaria, and Spain. These countries' climate and soil conditions are ideal for growing high-quality lavender, producing superior essential oil.

## Uses

1. **Stress Relief and Relaxation:** Lavender's calming aroma helps to reduce stress, anxiety, and tension, promoting relaxation and overall well-being.
2. **Sleep Support:** Its soothing properties make it an excellent aid for improving sleep quality and combating insomnia.
3. **Skin Health:** Lavender's antimicrobial and anti-inflammatory properties help to soothe irritated skin, promote wound healing, and minimize the appearance of scars and blemishes.
4. **Pain Relief:** Lavender can help alleviate headaches, muscle aches, and joint pain when used in massage or topical applications.

## Aromatherapy Recipes

**1. Relaxing Diffuser Blend:**
- 4 drops of Lavender essential oil
- drops of Bergamot essential oil
- 1 drop Ylang Ylang essential oil

Combine the oils in your diffuser and enjoy the calming and uplifting aroma.

**2. Sleep-Promoting Pillow Spray:**
- 1 oz distilled water
- 1 oz witch hazel
- 10 drops of Lavender essential oil

Mix the ingredients in a small spray bottle, and spritz them onto your pillow before bedtime to encourage restful sleep.

**3. Soothing Skin Serum:**
- 1 oz Jojoba oil
- 5 drops of Lavender essential oil
- 3 drops Frankincense essential oil
- 2 drops of Tea Tree essential oil

Combine the oils in a dark glass bottle and gently shake to mix. Apply a few drops to clean the skin, focusing on irritation, blemishes, or scarring areas.

**4. Lavender-infused Massage Oil:**
- 4 oz Sweet Almond oil
- 20 drops of Lavender essential oil

Mix the oils in a dark glass bottle and use the blend as a massage oil to help alleviate muscle tension and joint pain and promote relaxation.

By incorporating lavender essential oil into your aromatherapy and skincare routine, you can benefit from its calming, soothing, and healing properties.

# Peppermint Essential Oil

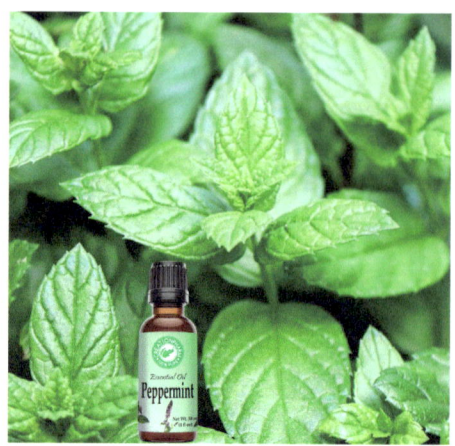

Peppermint essential oil is derived from the Mentha x piperita or menta x Piperita arvensis plant leaves. This refreshing and versatile oil is widely used in aromatherapy and various applications for its numerous therapeutic properties. Peppermint's cooling, stimulating, and soothing effects make it a popular choice for multiple purposes.

## Aroma Description

Peppermint essential oil has a strong, fresh, and minty aroma with a slightly sweet undertone. Its cooling and refreshing scent can energize and uplift the mood.

## Countries of Origin

Peppermint is primarily cultivated in several countries, with the most prominent ones being the United States, India, and various countries in Europe. These regions' climate and soil conditions are ideal for growing high-quality peppermint, producing superior essential oil.

## Uses

1. **Focus and Mental Clarity:** Peppermint's stimulating properties can help improve concentration, alertness, and cognitive function.
2. **Headache Relief:** Inhaling peppermint essential oil or applying it topically (diluted) can help alleviate headaches and migraines.
3. **Digestive Support:** Peppermint oil can help ease digestive discomfort, including indigestion, bloating, and nausea.
4. **Respiratory Health:** Its cooling and decongestant effects make it helpful in relieving nasal congestion and supporting overall respiratory health.

## Aromatherapy Recipes

**1. Focus-Enhancing Diffuser Blend:**
- 4 drops Peppermint essential oil
- 3 drops Rosemary essential oil
- 2 drops of Lemon essential oil

Combine the oils in your diffuser and enjoy the refreshing and invigorating aroma that promotes focus and mental clarity.

## 2. Headache-Relief Roll-On:
- 10 ml Jojoba oil
- 5 drops Peppermint essential oil
- 3 drops Lavender essential oil
- 2 drops Eucalyptus essential oil

Combine the oils in a 10 ml roll-on bottle and gently shake to mix. Apply to temples, forehead, and the back of the neck when experiencing headaches.

## 3. Digestive Support Massage Oil:
- 2 oz Sweet Almond oil
- 8 drops Peppermint essential oil
- 4 drops of Ginger essential oil
- 4 drops of Fennel essential oil

Mix the oils in a dark glass bottle and apply the blend as a massage oil to the abdomen to help alleviate digestive discomfort.

## 1. Congestion-Relief Chest Rub:
- 1 oz Coconut oil
- 5 drops Peppermint essential oil
- 5 drops of Eucalyptus essential oil
- 3 drops Rosemary essential oil

Mix the oils in a small jar and gently massage the blend onto the chest to help relieve nasal congestion and support respiratory health.

# Eucalyptus Essential Oil

Eucalyptus essential oil is extracted from the leaves of the Eucalyptus globulus tree, a native Australian plant known for its many therapeutic properties. In aromatherapy, eucalyptus oil is particularly valued for its benefits to respiratory health and the immune system and its ability to clear congestion and ease coughs.

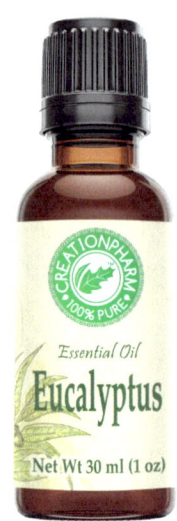

## Aroma Description

Eucalyptus essential oil has a fresh, crisp, and invigorating aroma with a robust and camphoraceous aroma and a hint of woodiness. Its refreshing and purifying fragrance makes it popular for various therapeutic applications.

## Countries of Origin

While Australia is the primary source of eucalyptus, the plant is also cultivated in favorable climates, such as China, India, Portugal, Spain, and South Africa. These regions provide the ideal conditions for growing high-quality eucalyptus, producing superior essential oil.

## Uses

1. **Respiratory Health:** Eucalyptus oil is well-known for supporting respiratory health by clearing congestion, easing coughs, and helping to reduce inflammation.
2. **Immune Support:** Its antimicrobial properties make it a practical choice for boosting the immune system and combating infections.
3. **Pain Relief:** Eucalyptus oil has analgesic and anti-inflammatory properties, making it helpful in relieving muscle and joint pain.
4. **Mental Clarity:** The refreshing aroma of eucalyptus oil can help improve focus and concentration.

## Aromatherapy Recipes

### 1. Respiratory Support Diffuser Blend:
- 4 drops of Eucalyptus essential oil
- 3 drops Peppermint essential oil
- 2 drops of Lavender essential oil

Combine the oils in your diffuser and enjoy the soothing aroma that promotes respiratory health and clear breathing.

### 1. Immune-Boosting Roll-On:
- 10 ml Jojoba oil
- 5 drops of Eucalyptus essential oil
- 4 drops of Tea Tree essential oil
- 3 drops of Lemon essential oil

Combine the oils in a 10 ml roll-on bottle and gently shake to mix. Apply to the wrists and behind the ears to support immune function.

### 2. Pain-Relieving Massage Oil:
- 2 oz Sweet Almond oil
- 8 drops of Eucalyptus essential oil
- 5 drops of Lavender essential oil
- 3 drops Rosemary essential oil

Mix the oils in a dark glass bottle and apply the blend as a massage oil to sore muscles and joints for pain relief.

### 3. Focus and Mental Clarity Inhaler:
- Aromatherapy inhaler
- 5 drops of Eucalyptus essential oil
- 4 drops of Rosemary essential oil
- 2 drops Peppermint essential oil

Add the essential oils to the cotton wick of an aromatherapy inhaler. Inhale the refreshing aroma whenever you need a mental boost or improved focus.

# Tea Tree Essential Oil

Tea tree essential oil, extracted from the leaves of the Melaleuca alternifolia plant, is highly prized for its potent antimicrobial properties. Tea tree oil is widely used in aromatherapy to address skin conditions, promote wound healing, and enhance household cleaning routines.

## Aroma Description

Tea tree essential oil has a fresh, medicinal, and slightly herbaceous aroma with a camphoraceous undertone. Its distinctive scent is invigorating and purifying, making it an excellent choice for various therapeutic and cleansing applications.

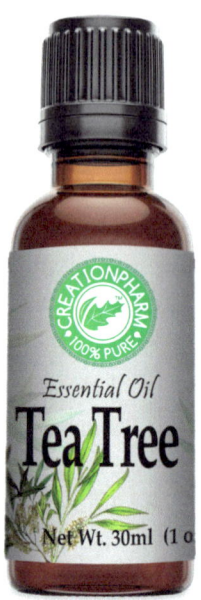

## Countries of Origin

The primary source of tea tree essential oil is Australia, where the Melaleuca alternifolia plant is native. Australia is renowned for producing high-quality tea tree oil due to its ideal climate and growing conditions.

## Uses

1. **Skin Care:** Tea tree oil's antimicrobial and anti-inflammatory properties effectively treat acne, soothing skin irritations and promoting wound healing.
2. **Immune Support:** The oil's powerful antiviral, antibacterial, and antifungal properties can help boost the immune system and combat infections.
3. **Respiratory Health:** Tea tree oil can help alleviate congestion and support respiratory health when inhaled.
4. **Household Cleaning:** Its antimicrobial properties make it a popular addition to natural cleaning products and disinfectants.

## Aromatherapy Recipes

**1. Acne Spot Treatment:**
- 1 tablespoon Aloe Vera gel
- 3 drops of Tea Tree essential oil

Combine the Aloe Vera gel and tea tree oil in a small container. Apply a small amount to the affected area using a cotton swab to help reduce inflammation and clear acne.

### 2. Immune-Boosting Diffuser Blend:
- 4 drops of Tea Tree essential oil
- 3 drops of Lemon essential oil
- 2 drops Eucalyptus essential oil

Combine the essential oils in your diffuser and enjoy the immune-boosting and purifying aroma.

### 3. Respiratory Relief Steam Inhalation:
- A bowl of hot water
- 2 drops of Tea Tree essential oil
- 2 drops of Eucalyptus essential oil

Add the essential oils to a bowl of hot water. Lean over the bowl with a towel draped over your head to trap the steam, and inhale deeply for 5-10 minutes to help relieve congestion and support respiratory health.

### 4. All-Purpose Household Cleaner:
- 16 oz spray bottle
- 1 cup distilled white vinegar
- 1 cup water
- 15 drops of Tea Tree essential oil
- 10 drops of Lemon essential oil

Combine the vinegar, water, and essential oils in a spray bottle. Shake well before each use and spray onto surfaces, wiping clean with a microfiber cloth for a natural, antimicrobial cleaning solution.

# Lemon Essential Oil

Lemon essential oil, derived from the rinds of Citrus limon fruit, is known for its uplifting and energizing properties. In aromatherapy, lemon oil is widely used to enhance mood, purify the air, and serve as a natural household cleaner.

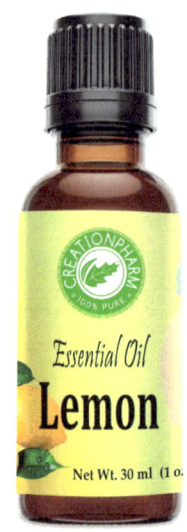

## Aroma Description

Lemon essential oil has a bright, tangy, refreshing citrus scent. Its aroma is invigorating and revitalizing, making it an excellent choice for boosting mood and energy levels and promoting mental clarity.

## Countries of Origin

Prominent countries for lemon essential oil include Italy, Spain, Argentina, and the United States, particularly California and Florida. These countries have ideal climates and growing conditions for cultivating high-quality lemon fruits for oil production.

## Uses

1. **Mood Enhancement:** Lemon oil's uplifting and energizing aroma can help improve mood and alleviate anxiety or stress.
2. **Air Purification:** The oil's antiviral and antibacterial properties effectively purify the air and neutralize unpleasant odors.
3. **Household Cleaning:** Lemon oil's natural disinfectant properties make it an excellent addition to homemade cleaning products.
4. **Skin Care:** Lemon essential oil can help brighten the skin and improve complexion when used in skincare routines. However, it is photosensitizing, so avoiding sun exposure after the application is essential.

## Aromatherapy Recipes

**1. Energizing Diffuser Blend:**
- 4 drops of Lemon essential oil
- 3 drops Peppermint essential oil
- 2 drops Rosemary essential oil

Combine the essential oils in your diffuser and enjoy the energizing and uplifting aroma.

## 2. Natural Air Freshener:
- 8 oz spray bottle
- 1 cup distilled water
- 10 drops of Lemon essential oil
- 5 drops of Lavender essential oil

Combine the water and essential oils in a spray bottle. Shake well before each use and spritz into the air to freshen and purify your living space.

## 3. All-Purpose Household Cleaner:
- 16 oz spray bottle
- 1 cup distilled white vinegar
- 1 cup water
- 15 drops of Lemon essential oil
- 10 drops of Tea Tree essential oil

Combine the vinegar, water, and essential oils in a spray bottle. Shake well before each use and spray onto surfaces, wiping clean with a microfiber cloth for a natural, antimicrobial cleaning solution.

## 4. Skin Brightening Toner:
- 4 oz spray bottle
- ¼ cup witch hazel
- ¼ cup distilled water
- 10 drops of Lemon essential oil
- 5 drops of Lavender essential oil

Combine the witch hazel, water, and essential oils in a spray bottle. Shake well before each use and mist onto clean skin, avoiding the eye area. Avoid sun exposure after application due to lemon oil's photosensitizing properties.

# Frankincense Essential Oil

Frankincense essential oil, derived from the resin of the Boswellia tree, has been cherished for centuries for its grounding and spiritual properties. In aromatherapy, frankincense is known to promote relaxation, support the immune system, and improve the appearance of the skin.

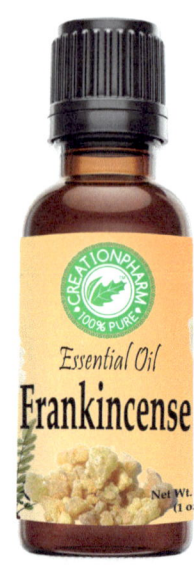

## Aroma Description

Frankincense essential oil has a rich, warm, and earthy aroma with hints of spice and sweetness. Its scent is often described as grounding and calming, making it perfect for meditation and relaxation.

## Countries of Origin

Prominent countries for frankincense essential oil include Oman, Somalia, Ethiopia, and India. These countries have the ideal climate and environmental conditions for the growth and cultivation of the Boswellia trees, which produce the resin used to create the oil.

## Uses

1. **Relaxation and Meditation:** The grounding and calming aroma of frankincense can support peace, reduce feelings of anxiety, and enhance meditation practices.
2. **Immune Support:** Frankincense oil has natural immune-boosting properties, which can help support overall health and well-being.
3. **Skin Care:** The oil is known for its ability to rejuvenate and improve the appearance of the skin, making it a popular choice for skincare routines and products.
4. **Emotional Balance:** Frankincense can help promote emotional balance and mental clarity, making it an excellent choice for stress relief and personal growth practices.

## Aromatherapy Recipes

### 1. Relaxing Diffuser Blend:
- 4 drops of Frankincense essential oil
- 3 drops Lavender essential oil
- 2 drops Ylang Ylang essential oil

Combine the essential oils in your diffuser and enjoy the soothing aroma.

## 2. Immune Support Roll-On:
- 10 ml roll-on bottle
- 2 tsp fractionated coconut oil
- 5 drops of Frankincense essential oil
- 5 drops of Lemon essential oil
- 3 drops of Tea Tree essential oil

Combine the essential oils and fractionated coconut oil in a roll-on bottle. Apply to the bottoms of the feet, wrists, or behind the ears to support immune health.

## 3. Rejuvenating Facial Serum:
- 1 oz glass dropper bottle
- 1 oz jojoba oil
- 6 drops of Frankincense essential oil
- 4 drops of Lavender essential oil
- 4 drops of Geranium essential oil

Combine the jojoba oil and essential oils in the dropper bottle. Apply a few drops to clean the skin, massaging gently in circular motions.

## 4. Grounding Meditation Mist:
- 4 oz spray bottle
- ¼ cup distilled water
- ¼ cup witch hazel
- 10 drops of Frankincense essential oil
- 5 drops Cedarwood essential oil

Combine the water, witch hazel, and essential oils in a spray bottle. Shake well before each use and mist around your meditation space or onto your body to promote relaxation and grounding.

# Rosemary Essential Oil

Rosemary essential oil, extracted from the leaves of the Rosmarinus officinalis plant, is known for its stimulating and invigorating properties. It is commonly used to help improve mental clarity, support memory, and promote healthy hair growth.

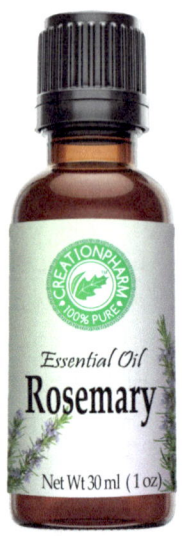

## Scent Description

Rosemary essential oil has a fresh, herbaceous, slightly woody aroma with a hint of camphor. Its refreshing scent is perfect for stimulating the mind and enhancing focus.

## Countries of Origin

Major countries for rosemary essential oil include Spain, Tunisia, Morocco, and France. These countries have the ideal climate and environmental conditions for the growth and cultivation of the Rosmarinus officinalis plant.

## Uses

1. **Mental Clarity and Focus:** The stimulating aroma of rosemary essential oil can help improve mental clarity and focus, making it an excellent choice for enhancing productivity and cognitive function.
2. **Memory Support:** Rosemary oil has been traditionally used for supporting memory and concentration.
3. **Hair Care:** The oil promotes healthy hair growth and reduces hair loss, making it a popular choice for hair care products and treatments.
4. **Muscle Tension Relief:** Rosemary oil has natural analgesic properties, making it helpful in relieving muscle tension and discomfort.

## Aromatherapy Recipes

**1. Focus and Clarity Diffuser Blend:**
- 5 drops of Rosemary essential oil
- 3 drops Peppermint essential oil
- 2 drops of Lemon essential oil

Combine the essential oils in your diffuser and enjoy the invigorating and focusing aroma.

## 2. Memory Support Inhaler:
- Aromatherapy inhaler
- 5 drops of Rosemary essential oil
- 4 drops of Basil essential oil
- 3 drops of Lemon essential oil

Add the essential oils to the aromatherapy inhaler and use them to support memory and concentration.

## 3. Hair Growth Scalp Massage Oil:
- 2 oz glass dropper bottle
- 2 oz jojoba oil
- 10 drops of Rosemary essential oil
- 5 drops of Lavender essential oil
- 5 drops Cedarwood essential oil

Combine the jojoba oil and essential oils in the dropper bottle. Apply a few drops to the scalp and massage gently to stimulate hair growth.

## 4. Muscle Tension Relief Massage Oil:
- 4 oz glass bottle
- 4 oz carrier oil (e.g., sweet almond oil or fractionated coconut oil)
- 15 drops of Rosemary essential oil
- 10 drops of Lavender essential oil
- 5 drops of Eucalyptus essential oil

Combine the carrier oil and essential oils in the bottle. Gently massage sore muscles and tension areas as needed for relief.

# Roman Chamomile Essential Oil

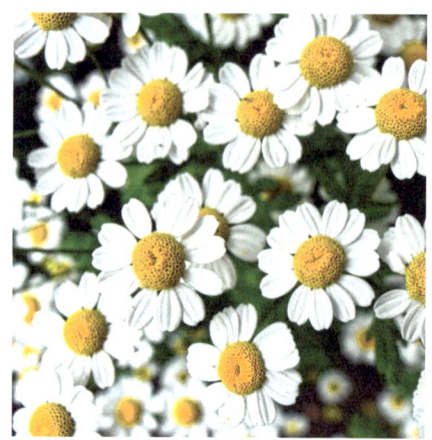

Roman chamomile essential oil, derived from the flowers of the Anthemis nobilis plant, is well-known for its gentle and soothing properties. It is ideal for calming the mind, easing stress, and supporting healthy sleep.

## Aroma Description

Roman chamomile essential oil has a sweet, herbaceous, and slightly fruity aroma with apple notes. Its gentle and soothing scent is comforting and calming, making it a popular choice for relaxation and stress relief.

## Countries of Origin

Prominent countries of origin for Roman chamomile essential oil include the United Kingdom, France, Belgium, and Italy. These regions offer the ideal climate and environmental conditions for the growth and cultivation of the Anthemis nobilis plant.

## Uses

1. **Stress Relief and Relaxation**: The calming properties of Roman chamomile oil make it excellent for stress relief and relaxation, helping to ease tension and promote a sense of inner peace.
2. **Sleep Support:** Roman chamomile is known for promoting restful sleep and is often used in bedtime routines to help individuals fall asleep more easily.
3. **Skin Care**: Roman chamomile oil's gentle, soothing nature makes it suitable for sensitive skin and various skin conditions, including redness and irritation.
4. **Emotional Balance**: The oil is frequently used to support emotional well-being and create inner harmony.

## Aromatherapy Recipes

### 1. Relaxation and Stress Relief Diffuser Blend:
- 4 drops Roman Chamomile essential oil
- 4 drops of Lavender essential oil
- 2 drops of Orange essential oil

Combine the essential oils in your diffuser and enjoy the calming and relaxing aroma.

## 2. Sleep Support Pillow Spray:
- 2 oz glass spray bottle
- 1 oz distilled water
- 1 oz witch hazel
- 10 drops Roman Chamomile essential oil
- 10 drops of Lavender essential oil

Combine the distilled water, witch hazel, and essential oils in the spray bottle. Shake well and spritz onto your pillow before bedtime to support restful sleep.

## 3. Skin Soother Serum:
- 1 oz glass dropper bottle
- 1 oz carrier oil (e.g., jojoba oil or sweet almond oil)
- 5 drops Roman Chamomile essential oil
- 5 drops of Lavender essential oil
- 3 drops Frankincense essential oil

Combine the carrier oil and essential oils in the dropper bottle. Apply a few drops to clean the skin and gently massage to soothe and moisturize.

## 4. Emotional Balance Rollerball Blend:
- 10 ml glass rollerball bottle
- Carrier oil (e.g., fractionated coconut oil or jojoba oil)
- 4 drops Roman Chamomile essential oil
- 4 drops of Bergamot essential oil
- 2 drops Frankincense essential oil

Add the essential oils to the rollerball bottle and fill the rest with your chosen carrier oil. Apply the blend to your wrists, temples, and behind the ears to promote emotional balance and inner harmony.

# Sweet Orange Essential Oil

Sweet orange essential oil is derived from the peel of the Citrus sinensis fruit and is known for its sweet, citrusy aroma. It is commonly used in aromatherapy for its uplifting, mood-enhancing properties and ability to reduce stress and act as a natural air freshener.

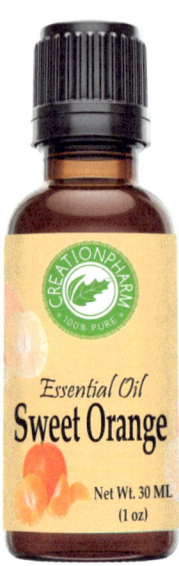

## Aroma Description

Sweet orange essential oil has a bright, sweet, and citrusy scent with a slightly tangy undertone. Its aroma is refreshing and uplifting and evokes happiness and warmth, making it a popular choice for mood enhancement and stress reduction.

## Countries of Origin

Prominent countries for sweet orange essential oil include Brazil, the United States (particularly Florida and California), Italy, and Spain. These regions have optimal climates and conditions for the growth and cultivation of Citrus sinensis trees.

## Uses

1. **Mood Enhancement**: Sweet orange essential oil is known for uplifting the mood and creating a positive atmosphere, making it an excellent choice for combating sadness or low energy.
2. **Stress Reduction**: The refreshing and uplifting aroma of sweet orange oil can help to reduce stress and promote a sense of calm and relaxation.
3. **Natural Air Freshener**: Due to its pleasant scent, the sweet orange essential oil is often used as a natural air freshener in homes and workplaces.
4. **Cleaning**: The oil also has antimicrobial properties, making it a popular addition to homemade cleaning solutions.

## Aromatherapy Recipes

**1. Uplifting Diffuser Blend:**
- 5 drops of Sweet Orange essential oil
- 3 drops Grapefruit essential oil
- 2 drops of Bergamot essential oil

Combine the essential oils in your diffuser and enjoy the bright, uplifting aroma.

**2. Stress-Reducing Rollerball Blend:**
- 10 ml glass rollerball bottle
- Carrier oil (e.g., fractionated coconut oil or jojoba oil)
- 5 drops of Sweet Orange essential oil
- 5 drops of Lavender essential oil
- 3 drops Ylang Ylang essential oil

Add the essential oils to the rollerball bottle and fill the rest with your chosen carrier oil. Apply the blend to your wrists, temples, and behind the ears to reduce stress and promote relaxation.

**3. Natural Air Freshener Spray:**
- 4 oz glass spray bottle
- 3 oz distilled water
- 1 oz witch hazel or vodka
- 20 drops of Sweet Orange essential oil
- 10 drops of Lemon essential oil
- 10 drops of Grapefruit essential oil

Combine the distilled water, witch hazel, vodka, and essential oils in the spray bottle. Shake well and use as needed to freshen the air in your home or workplace.

**4. Homemade All-Purpose Cleaner:**
- 16 oz glass spray bottle
- 14 oz distilled water
- 2 oz white vinegar
- 20 drops of Sweet Orange essential oil
- 10 drops of Tea Tree essential oil

Combine the distilled water, white vinegar, and essential oils in the spray bottle. Shake well and use it to clean various home surfaces, such as countertops, sinks, and appliances.

# Ylang-Ylang Essential Oil

Ylang-ylang essential oil is derived from the flowers of the Cananga odorata tree, known for its exotic, sweet, and floral aroma. It is commonly used in aromatherapy for its calming and stress-relieving effects and its ability to promote emotional balance and well-being.

## Aroma Description

Ylang-ylang essential oil has a rich, sweet, and floral scent with slightly fruity undertones. Its intoxicating and sensual aroma can help evoke feelings of relaxation and tranquility, making it an excellent choice for calming the mind and reducing stress.

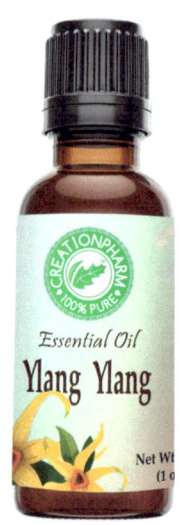

## Countries of Origin

Prominent countries of origin for ylang-ylang essential oil include Madagascar, the Comoros Islands, the Philippines, and Indonesia. These regions have the ideal climate and conditions for the growth and cultivation of the Cananga odorata tree.

## Uses

1. **Calming and Stress Relief:** Ylang-ylang essential oil is known for its ability to manage the mind, reduce stress, and promote relaxation, making it a popular choice for those seeking emotional balance.
2. **Emotional Balance:** The sweet, floral aroma of ylang-ylang can help create a soothing atmosphere that fosters emotional balance and well-being.
3. **Skincare:** Ylang-ylang oil is known for its ability to balance skin oil production, making it a beneficial addition to skincare routines, particularly for those with combination or oily skin.
4. **Aphrodisiac:** The sensual aroma of ylang-ylang is often used to enhance romantic and intimate settings.

## Aromatherapy Recipes

**1. Relaxing Diffuser Blend**:
- 4 drops Ylang Ylang essential oil
- 3 drops Lavender essential oil
- 2 drops Cedarwood essential oil

Combine the essential oils in your diffuser and enjoy the calming and relaxing aroma.

### 2. Emotional Balance Rollerball Blend:
- 10 ml glass rollerball bottle
- Carrier oil (e.g., fractionated coconut oil or jojoba oil)
- 5 drops Ylang Ylang essential oil
- 4 drops of Bergamot essential oil
- 3 drops Frankincense essential oil

Add the essential oils to the rollerball bottle and fill the rest with your chosen carrier oil. Apply the blend to your wrists, temples, and behind the ears to promote emotional balance and well-being.

### 3. Sensual Massage Oil:
- 2 oz carrier oil (e.g., sweet almond oil or grapeseed oil)
- 6 drops Ylang Ylang essential oil
- 4 drops of Patchouli essential oil
- 4 drops of Sandalwood essential oil

Mix the carrier oil and essential oils in a glass bottle. Use as a massage oil to enhance intimacy and relaxation.

### 4. Balancing Facial Serum:
- 1 oz jojoba oil
- 3 drops Ylang Ylang essential oil
- 3 drops of Geranium essential oil
- 2 drops of Lavender essential oil

Combine the jojoba oil and essential oils in a glass bottle and mix well. Apply a few drops of the serum to your face after cleansing and toning, focusing on areas with excess oil production.

Chapter Four

# Herbs and Plants for Essential Oil Production

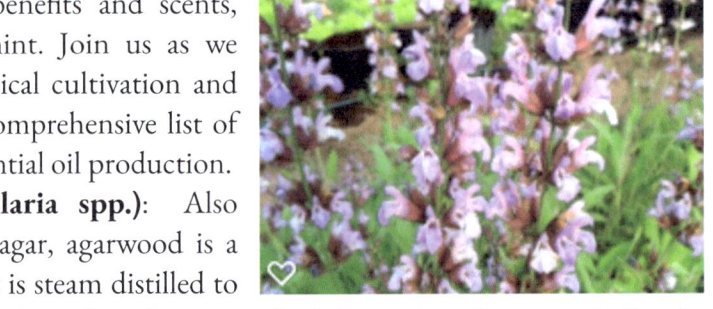

Discover the power of essential oils! Many plants offer unique therapeutic benefits and scents, from lavender to peppermint. Join us as we explore sustainable and ethical cultivation and harvesting practices for a comprehensive list of aromatic plants used in essential oil production.

1. **Agarwood (Aquilaria spp.)**: Also known as oud or agar, agarwood is a resinous wood that is steam distilled to produce a rich, woody, and earthy essential oil. It is primarily grown in Southeast Asia and requires a unique fungal infection to develop the resin that is used to make the oil.
2. **Blue Tansy (Tanacetum annuum)**: This plant produces a striking blue oil that has a sweet, floral scent. It is native to Morocco and requires a specific distillation process to extract the oil without causing discoloration.
3. **Helichrysum (Helichrysum italicum)**: This plant, also known as immortelle, produces an oil with a warm, herbaceous scent. It is commonly used for skin care and requires a large amount of botanical matter to produce a small amount of oil.
4. **Palo Santo (Bursera graveolens)**: This tree native to South America produces a wood that is used for incense and is also steam distilled to produce essential oil with an aroma considered sweet, woody, and citrusy.
5. **Spikenard (Nardostachys jatamansi)**: This plant, native to the Himalayas, produces an oil with a musky, earthy, and grounding scent. It has been used for thousands of years in Ayurvedic medicine and requires a lengthy distillation process.
6. **Ylang Ylang (Cananga odorata)**: This tree, native to Southeast Asia, produces a flower that is steam distilled to produce an essential oil with a floral, sweet and exotic aroma. It is commonly used in perfumes and requires careful harvesting to ensure the quality of the oil.

# A Comprehensive List of Aromatic Plants and Their Properties

There are numerous plants and herbs used to produce essential oils, each with distinct properties and applications. While it's impossible to cover every single plant here, we provide an overview of some common and lesser-known aromatic plants:

1. **Basil (Ocimum basilicum)**: Basil essential oil is revered for its energizing and uplifting influences. It is often used to alleviate mental fatigue, improve focus, and ease muscle tension.
2. **Bergamot (Citrus bergamia)**: Bergamot essential oil is prized for its uplifting and calming effects. It can help alleviate stress, anxiety, and depression, and is also known for its antimicrobial properties.
3. **Cedarwood (Cedrus atlantica)**: Cedarwood essential oil with it's grounding and calming aroma, makes it ideal for stress relief and promoting relaxation. It also supports respiratory health and is often used in skincare products for its soothing and astringent properties.
4. **Clary Sage (Salvia sclarea)**: Clary sage essential oil is calming, relaxing, and is often used to ease stress, anxiety, and menstrual discomfort. It also has a reputation for promoting hormonal balance and supporting women's health.
5. **Cypress (Cupressus sempervirens)**: Cypress essential oil is beneficial for respiratory health and is often used to help clear congestion and ease breathing. It also has astringent and antispasmodic properties, making it useful for skincare and muscle pain relief.
6. **Geranium (Pelargonium graveolens)**: Geranium essential oil is commonly used for its balancing and soothing properties. It supports emotional well-being and is often used in skincare products for to regulate oil production and promoting clearer, healthy skin.
7. **Ginger (Zingiber officinale)**: Ginger essential is often used to relieve digestive discomfort, ease nausea, and support circulation and is warming and stimulating. It can also provide relief from muscle and joint pain.
8. **Grapefruit (Citrus paradisi)**: Grapefruit essential oil is touted for its uplifting, energizing effects. It is commonly used to help combat fatigue, uplift mood, and support weight management by curbing cravings and promoting metabolism.
9. **Helichrysum (Helichrysum italicum)**: Helichrysum essential oil is prized for its powerful skin rejuvenating and healing properties. It is often used in skincare formulations for reducing the signs of aging and appearance of scars, wrinkles, and other skin issues.

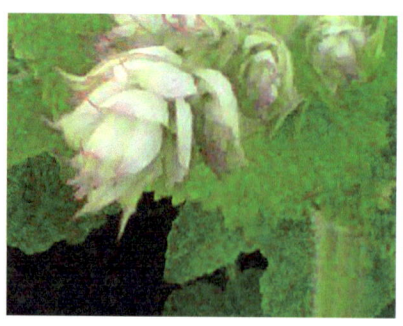

10. **Jasmine (Jasminum grandiflorum)**: Jasmine essential oil has intoxicating floral aroma with calming, uplifting properties. It is often used to alleviate stress, anxiety, and depression, and is also considered an aphrodisiac.

11. **Juniper Berry (Juniperus communis)**: Juniper berry essential oil is often used for its detoxifying and diuretic properties. It can support urinary and digestive health and is also used to alleviate muscle and joint pain.

12. **Lemongrass (Cymbopogon citratus)**: Lemongrass essential oil is considered an invigorating and refreshing aroma. It is often used to relieve muscle pain, repel insects, and support healthy digestion.

13. **Marjoram (Origanum majorana)**: Marjoram essential oil is warming and calming. Often used to support healthy digestion, alleviate muscle and joint pain, and promote relaxation and sleep.

14. **Myrrh (Commiphora myrrha)**: Myrrh essential oil is considered to have soothing and healing properties. It is quite often used to support oral health, promote clear skin, and ease respiratory issues.

15. **Neroli (Citrus aurantium)**: Neroli essential oil is prized for its uplifting and calming effects. It is a go to aroma used to relax stress, anxiety, and depression, and is particularly beneficial for skincare for mature or sensitive skin.

16. **Patchouli (Pogostemon cablin)**: Patchouli essential oil has a somewhat earthy, sweet but pungent aroma and grounding properties. It is often used in perfumes and skincare products to promote healthy skin, and believed by many to reduce the appearance of scars, wrinkles, and blemishes. Patchouli also has a calming effect and can help alleviate stress and anxiety.

17. **Roman Chamomile (Chamaemelum nobile)**: Roman chamomile essential oil is asoothing and calming aroma. It is often used to ease stress, anxiety, and promote relaxation, especially before sleep. Roman chamomile is also helpful in soothing irritated skin and reducing inflammation.

18. **Sandalwood (Santalum album)**: Sandalwood essential oil is revered for its calming, grounding properties and its rich, woody aroma. It is often used in meditation and spiritual practices for its ability to promote inner peace and clarity. Sandalwood oil is also beneficial for skincare, particularly for dry or aging skin, as it helps to soothe and moisturize.

19. **Vetiver (Vetiveria zizanioides)**: Vetiver essential oil has deep earthy almost sharp aroma and grounding effects. It is often used to promote relaxation, ease anxiety, and support emotional balance. Vetiver oil is also beneficial for skincare, as it can support your overall skin health helping to reduce scar and blemish visuals.

# Cultivation and Harvesting Practices

Cultivating and harvesting practices have a significant impact on the quality and therapeutic value of essential oils. The following factors play are important criteria for the production of the highest quality oils:

- **Soil quality:** Healthy soil provides the necessary nutrients for plants to thrive and produce the desired aromatic compounds.
- **Climate and environmental factors:** Different plants have specific climate and environmental requirements for optimal growth and essential oil production.
- **Harvesting time:** The timing of harvesting can greatly influence the quality and composition of essential oils. Factors such as time of day, season, and plant maturity should be considered.
- **Harvesting methods:** Careful handling of plants during harvest can preserve the delicate aromatic compounds and prevent damage that could negatively affect the quality of the essential oils.

# Sustainability and Ethical Sourcing of Essential Oils

As the demand for essential oils grows, it's vital to consider the sustainability and ethical sourcing of these precious resources. Here are some key aspects to consider when choosing essential oils:

- **Sustainable farming practices:** Look for companies that prioritize sustainable farming practices, such as organic cultivation, water conservation, and soil preservation.
- **Ethical sourcing and fair trade:** Support companies that ensure fair wages, safe working conditions, and equitable treatment for the farmers and distillers involved in essential oil production.
- **Endangered or overharvested species:** Be cautious about using essential oils derived from endangered or overharvested plants, such as rosewood or sandalwood. Opt for alternatives or sustainably sourced options when possible.
- **Transparency and traceability:** Choose companies that provide detailed information about the source, cultivation, and production of their essential oils, as well as third-party testing for quality and purity.

Chapter Five

# Methods of Aromatherapy

Aromatherapy methods refer to how essential oils can promote health and well-being. There are various aromatherapy methods, including inhalation, topical application, and internal use. Understanding the different ways of aromatherapy and their specific benefits can help you choose the best approach for your individual needs.

## Inhalation: Diffusers, Steam Inhalation, and Sprays

Inhalation is a popular method for using essential oils, as it allows their aroma and therapeutic properties to be quickly absorbed into the body. It can be achieved through diffusers, steam inhalation, and sprays. Diffusers disperse essential oils into the air, while steam inhalation involves adding essential oils to hot water and inhaling the steam. Another convenient way to apply essential oils to the air or surfaces is with sprays and misters. Each inhalation method has its benefits and can be tailored to specific needs.

## Topical Applications: Massage, Compresses, and Baths

Topical applications of essential oils involve applying them directly to the skin or incorporating them into massage oils, compresses, or baths. This method allows for targeted relief of physical discomfort, relaxation, and skin nourishment. Essential oils are absorbed through the skin and they can also have systemic effects, making it a popular method for therapeutic use.

# Internal Use: Safety and Guidelines

Internal use of essential oils refers to consuming or using them orally in cooking. While some essential oils may be safe for internal use, others can be toxic and cause adverse reactions. It is crucial to use caution and follow safety guidelines when using essential oils internally, including diluting them properly, using high-quality oils, and consulting a healthcare professional before use.

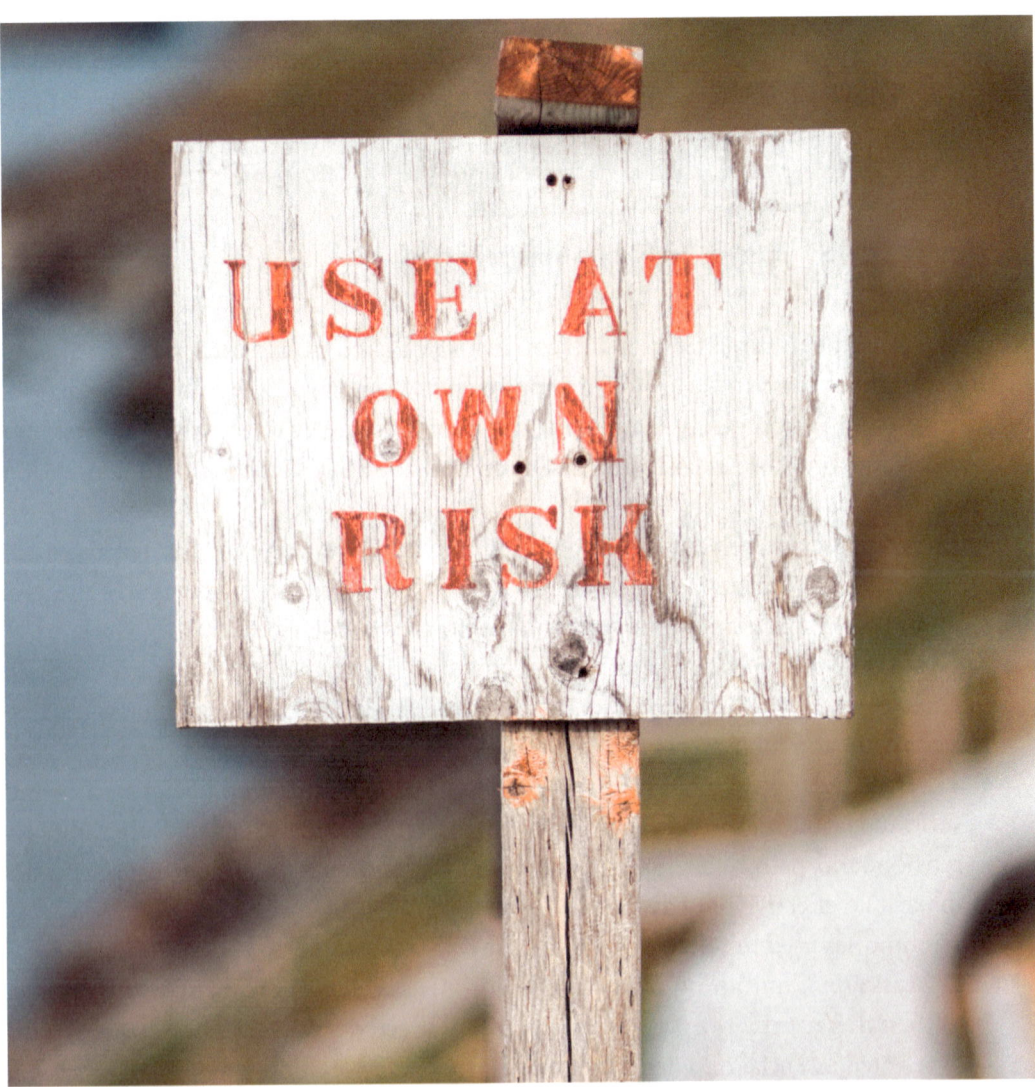

Chapter Six

# Aromatherapy for Physical Well-being

Aromatherapy has been used for centuries to promote physical health and well-being. This chapter will explore how essential oils can support natural healing processes in the body and asoothe various physical ailments. Aromatherapy offers a natural and holistic approach to physical wellness, from headaches to muscle pain and respiratory and digestive problems.

# Pain Relief and Inflammation

Aromatherapy, the therapeutic use of essential oils extracted from plants, has gained popularity recently as a natural and holistic approach to managing pain and inflammation. Numerous essential oils claim analgesic and anti-inflammatory effects that help remove discomfort and promote relaxation. Essential Oils for Pain Relief and Inflammation include:

- **Eucalyptus:** Known for its invigorating and refreshing aroma, eucalyptus essential oil is fairly analgesic and an anti-inflammatory agent. It is particularly effective in relieving muscle and joint pain and respiratory congestion.
- **Ginger:** With its warm and spicy scent, the ginger essential oil is an excellent choice for reducing inflammation and discomfort. It can help soothe muscle aches, joint pain, and menstrual cramps.
- **Lavender:** A popular choice in aromatherapy, the essential oil has a calming and soothing effect on the mind and body. An effective remedy for headaches, muscle tension, and pain relief, Its analgesic qualities and anti-inflammatory properties make it an effective remedy.

The techniques used in relieving pain are the following:

1. **Massage:** Combining essential oils with massage is an excellent way to deliver their therapeutic properties directly to the affected area. Mix a few drops of your selected essential oil with a carrier oils, such as sweet almond or jojoba, massaging the blend into the painful or inflamed areas. This method helps relieve pain, improves circulation, and promotes relaxation.
2. **Compresses:** A warm or cold compress using essential oils can immediately relieve various pain types. Add a few drops of essential oils to a vessel of warm or

cold water, soak a clean cloth in it and apply it to the painful area. The temperature of the compress will depend on the nature of the pain; for instance, warm compresses are suitable for soothing muscle aches, while cold compresses can help reduce inflammation and swelling.
3. **Topical Blends:** Creating a topical blend with essential oils and a carrier oil can offer targeted pain relief. Mix a few drops essential oil with a carrier oil and apply it directly. Topical blends are beneficial for addressing localized pain, such as joint discomfort or muscle soreness.

# Immune Support and Fighting Infections

A robust immune system is the cornerstone of good health, as it helps protect the body from illness and infections. Essential oils can be a valuable addition to your daily lifestyle to boost immune function and keep you feeling your best. Essential Oils for Immune Support and Fighting Infections are the following:

- **Tea Tree:** This oil has powerful antiseptic, antibacterial, and antiviral properties. Tea Tree essential oil is very effective in supporting the immune system and combating infections. It can help prevent and treat many ailments, from common colds to skin infections.
- **Oregano:** Oregano essential oil has potent antimicrobial and antiviral properties, making it an excellent choice for boosting immune function and fighting infections. It is instrumental in combating respiratory infections and can help alleviate symptoms of colds and flu. Oregano is very powerful. When using Oregano, research the proper dilution ratio to avoid potential severe burn-like irritations.
- **Lemon:** With its refreshing and uplifting scent, lemon essential oil is a very often selected choice for aromatherapy and a powerful immune booster. Its high concentration of vitamin C and antioxidant properties can help protect the body from harmful pathogens and support overall immune function.

Tips for incorporating essential oils into your daily routine:
1. **Diffusion:** Diffusing essential oils into the air is a simple yet effective way to harness their immune-boosting properties. Add a few drops of essential oil to a diffuser and let the aroma fill your living space. Diffusing essential oils like tea tree, Oregano, or lemon can help purify the air, reduce the spread of germs, and support overall immune function.
2. **Inhalation**: Inhaling essential oils can provide immediate immune support and help prevent the onset of illness. Place a couple drops of your selected essential oil on a tissue or cotton ball and inhale deeply for several breaths. This method

is particularly effective for respiratory infections and can relieve congestion and other cold symptoms.
3. **Topical Application:** Diluting essential oils with carrier oil and by applying them to the skin can offer targeted immune support. Mix a few drops of the essential oil with a carrier oil, such as Evening Primrose or jojoba, and apply it to the bottom of your feet, wrist, or upper chest. This method allows the oils to be absorbed through the skin entering the bloodstream, providing immune-boosting benefits.
4. **Household Cleaning:** Incorporating essential oils into your household cleaning routine can help create a healthier living environment and support immune function. Add a few drops of essential oils like lemon, tea tree, or oregano to a spray bottle, fill with water and use it as a natural surface cleaner. It not only disinfects surfaces but also fills your home with a pleasant, immune-supporting aroma.

# Respiratory Health

Essential oils can be pivotal in supporting respiratory health and addressing common issues such as allergies, colds, and congestion. With their natural, therapeutic properties, essential oils can provide relief and promote overall respiratory well-being.

Essential oils for Respiratory Health are the following:

- **Eucalyptus:** This essential oil is widely recognized for alleviating respiratory issues with its refreshing and invigorating aroma. Its potent expectorant and decongestant properties can help relieve nasal congestion, sinusitis, and symptoms associated with colds and flu.
- **Peppermint:** Peppermint essential oil is an excellent choice for supporting respiratory health and has cooling, soothing effects. The menthol content can help ease breathing difficulties, alleviate inflammation, and reduce symptoms of allergies and their ensuing respiratory infections.
- **Rosemary:** Rosemary essential oil ha stimulating, invigorating properties, indicating it beneficial for respiratory health. It can help reduce congestion, soothe respiratory discomfort, and alleviate symptoms related to bronchitis and asthma.

Methods for using essential oils to support respiratory health:
1. **Diffusers:** Using an aromatherapy diffuser to disperse essential oils into the atmosphere of any locale is a simple and effective way to support respiratory health. Add a few drops of your selected essential oil, such as eucalyptus, peppermint, or rosemary, to a diffuser, allowing the aroma to fill your living space. This method can help purify the air, reduce airborne allergens, and relieve respiratory discomfort.

2. **Steam Inhalation:** Steam inhalation is a powerful way to harness the therapeutic properties of essential oils and provide direct relief to the respiratory system. Fill a vessel with hot water and add a few drops of essential oil. Use a towel over your head and leaning over the bowl, inhale the aromatic steam for several minutes. This method is particularly effective for relieving congestion, sinusitis, and other respiratory issues.
3. **Personal Inhalers:** Personal inhalers, also known as aromatherapy inhalers or nasal inhalers, are portable devices that allow you to enjoy the potential benefits of essential oils when you are on the go. Add a few drops of essential oil to the inhaler's wick or cotton pad, and inhale as needed. This method provides targeted support for respiratory health and can be especially helpful during allergy season or when experiencing cold symptoms.

## Skin and Hair Care

Essential oils are a versatile and natural addition to your skin and hair care regimen. With their unique properties, essential oils can help address various skin and hair concerns, promoting overall health and well-being. Essential oils for skin and hair care:

- **Lavender:** A popular choice for skin healing, Lavender essential oil is known for its calming and soothing properties, making it. Its anti-inflammatory and antimicrobial properties can help reduce redness and irritation and promote healing in damaged skin. Additionally, lavender oil can condition hair, soothe the scalp, and promote hair growth.
- **Tea Tree:** Tea tree essential oil is revered for its powerful antiseptic, antimicrobial properties. It is especially beneficial for acne-prone skin and can help reduce inflammation, redness, and blemishes. For hair care, tea tree oil can address dandruff, soothe itchy scalp, and reduce excess oil production.
- **Rosemary:** Rosemary essential oil is stimulating and invigorating, making it an excellent choice for hair care. It can help promote hair growth, improve scalp health, and add shine to dull hair. Rosemary oil is also beneficial for the skin and can help improve circulation and combat signs of aging.

Incorporating essential oils into your skin and hair care routines:

1. **DIY Facial Serums:** Create a customized facial serum by adding a few drops of your appropriate skin care essential oil, such as lavender or tea tree, to a carrier oil like jojoba or Red Raspberyy oil. Apply this serum to your face after cleansing and toning to help address specific skin concerns and maintain a healthy complexion.

2. **Body Lotions:** Boost the benefits of your body lotion: add a few drops of essential oil, like lavender, before applying it to your skin. It can help soothe irritation, promote skin healing, and provide an aromatic experience during your daily skincare routine.
3. **Hair Treatments:** Enhance your hair care routine by incorporating essential oils, such as tea tree or rosemary, into your shampoo, conditioner, or hair mask. It can help address hair concerns like dandruff, promote growth, and improve overall health.

For example, create a DIY hair growth treatment by mixing a few drops of rosemary essential oil with a carrier oil. Massage this blend into your scalp, leave it on for at least 20 minutes, and then wash and rinse your hair as usual.

# Digestive Health

Aromatherapy can provide valuable support for digestive health by addressing common issues such as indigestion, bloating, and nausea. Essential oils, with their natural therapeutic properties, can help promote healthy digestion and alleviate digestive discomfort. In this section, we will explore essential oils like ginger, fennel, and peppermint that can improve digestive health and provide tips on using these oils in various application methods.

Essential Oils for Digestive Health
- **Ginger:** Ginger essential oil is warming and stimulating and is beneficial for digestion. It can help ease indigestion, reduce bloating, and alleviate nausea. Ginger oil is also known to support healthy digestion by proper absorption of nutrients through stimulating the digestive system.
- **Fennel:** Fennel essential oil is know to have antispasmodic and carminative effects, making it a viable alternative for addressing digestive issues. It can help relieve gas, bloating, and abdominal discomfort and promote regular bowel movements.
- **Peppermint:** Peppermint essential oil is known for its cooling and soothing effects, which can be helpful for digestion. It can help alleviate symptoms of indigestion, reduce gas and bloating, and relieve nausea.

Application Methods for Digestive Health
1. **Topical Application:** To use essential oils for digestive support, dilute them with an appropriate carrier oil such as coconut MCT or jojoba oil, before applying them to the skin. Gently massage the diluted essential oil onto your abdomen area to help relieve digestive discomfort and promote healthy diges-

tion. Follow proper dilution guidelines and perform a patch test to ensure skin compatibility.
2. **Aromatherapy Inhalation:** Inhaling essential oils can also provide digestive benefits. Use a diffuser to disperse your chosen essential oil, such as ginger or peppermint, into the air. Alternatively, add drops of essential oils to a cotton ball or tissues and inhale the aroma deeply. This method can help alleviate nausea and support overall digestive health.
3. **Warm Compress:** For an additional soothing effect, create a warm compress by adding a few drops of the appropriate essential oil, like fennel, to a vessel of warm water. Soaking a clean cloth in the water, wringing it out, and then placing it on your abdomen for 10-15 minutes. This method can help provide relief from abdominal discomfort and promote relaxation.

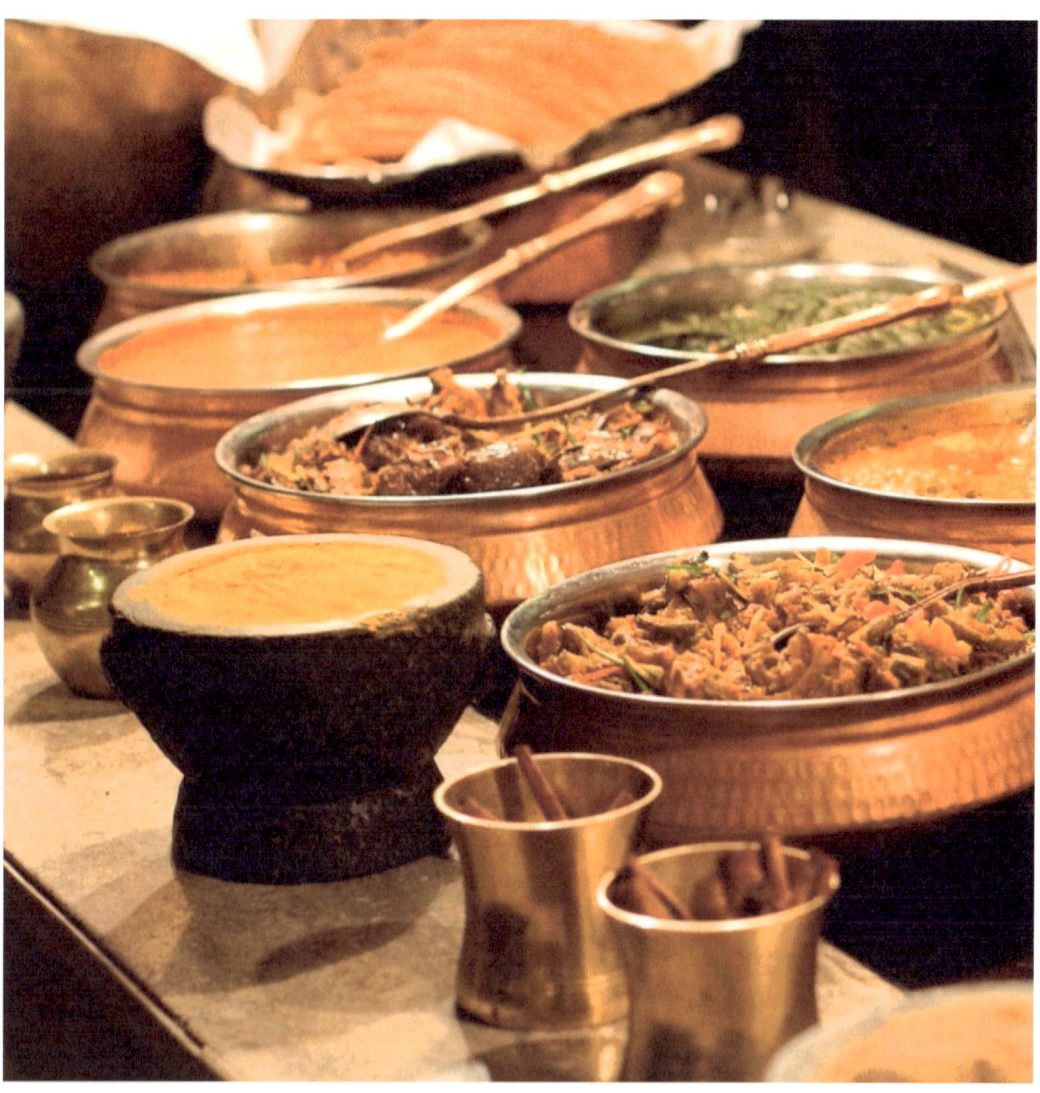

Chapter Seven

# Aromatherapy for Emotional and Mental Balance

Aromatherapy has long been used as a natural and holistic approach to supporting emotional and mental well-being. Essential oils have unique chemical compositions that can positively affect mood, reduce stress and anxiety, and promote relaxation. This section will explore the use of essential oils for emotional and mental balance, including their benefits, applications, and blending techniques.

## Stress and Anxiety Relief

In today's fast-paced world, stress and anxiety are common challenges. Aromatherapy can be an effective tool in managing these issues by promoting relaxation and mental clarity. This section will explore essential oils known for their calming properties, such as lavender, chamomile, and bergamot, and explain how to use them in various applications for stress relief and anxiety management.

1. **Diffusion:** Diffusing calming essential oils in your living or work environment help with creating a relaxing atmosphere that reduces stress and anxiety. Add a few drops of lavender, bergamot, or chamomile essential oil to your diffuser and let the soothing scents fill the room.
2. **Topical Application:** Dilute calming essential oils with a carrier oils like almond, coconut, or jojoba and apply them to pulse points like your wrists, temples, and behind your ears. It can help you experience the calming effects of the oils throughout the day. For instance, mix a few drops of lavender essential oil with carrier oil and gently massage it into your skin a while to relieve tension.
3. **Aromatherapy Bath:** Try adding a few drops of calming essential oils to your bathwater along with Epsom salts and/or carrier oil, to create a soothing and relaxing bath experience. Lavender, chamomile, and bergamot essential oils can help relieve stress and anxiety while you soak in the tub.
4. **Aromatherapy Massage:** Combine calming essential oils with carrier oil to create a relaxing massage oil. A gentle massage with lavender, chamomile, or

bergamot essential oils can help ease tension, reduce stress, and promote overall relaxation.
5. **Inhalation:** Inhaling calming essential oils can provide instant stress relief and help soothe anxiety. Place a few drops of the appropriate essential oil onto a tissue or cotton ball and inhale deeply, or add the oil to a personal inhaler or aromatherapy necklace for on-the-go stress relief.
6. **Pillow Mist:** Create a calming pillow mist by combining lavender, chamomile, or bergamot essential oil in a few drops blend with distilled water in a spray bottle. Mist your pillow and bedding before sleep to help promote relaxation and reduce nighttime anxiety.
7. **Aromatherapy Candles:** Light an aromatherapy candle scented with calming essential oils to create a peaceful atmosphere in your home. Lavender, chamomile, and bergamot-scented candles can help reduce stress and anxiety while providing a gentle, soothing fragrance.

# Mood Enhancement and Emotional Support

Essential oils can help support emotional well-being by stimulating positive emotions and uplifting the spirit. This section will discuss essential oils known for their mood-enhancing properties, such as citrus, jasmine, and rose, and methods for incorporating them into your daily routine to promote a sense of joy and emotional balance.
1. **Diffusion:** Use a diffuser to distribute mood-enhancing essential oil aromas throughout your living and work environment can help create an uplifting atmosphere. Add a few drops of citrus oils like lemon, orange, grapefruit, or floral oils like jasmine or rose to your diffuser and enjoy the cheerful and refreshing scents.
2. **Topical Application:** Dilute mood-enhancing essential oil with carrier oils and apply them to pulse points like your wrists, temples, and behind your ears. It allows the uplifting scents to be absorbed into your skin and provide emotional support throughout the day. For instance, mix a few drops of jasmine essential oil with carrier oil and massage gently into your skin to bring feelings of joy and happiness.
3. **Aromatherapy Shower:** Transform your daily shower into an uplifting experience by the addition of a few drops of mood enhancing essential oils to a washcloth or shower gel. Breathe in the refreshing scents of citrus or floral oils as the steam releases its aroma.
4. **Inhalation:** Inhaling mood-enhancing essential oils can provide an instant emotional boost. Place a few drops of the appropriate essential oil(s) on a tissue

or cotton ball and inhale deeply. Add the oil to a personal inhaler or aromatherapy necklace for on-the-go emotional support.
5. **Aromatherapy Massage:** Combine mood-enhancing essential oils with carrier oil to create an uplifting massage oil. A gentle massage with citrus or floral oils can help elevate your mood and promote emotional balance.
6. **Room Spray:** Create an uplifting room spray by combining a few drops essential oils like lemon, orange, or rose with distilled water in a spray bottle for mood enhancement. Use this spray to refresh your living space and encourage a positive atmosphere.
7. **Mood-Boosting Blend:** Experiment with creating personalized essential oil blends that cater to your emotional needs. Combine mood-enhancing oils like citrus and floral oils with grounding oils like cedarwood or vetiver to create a balanced, emotionally supportive blend.

# Sleep and Relaxation

A good night's sleep is important for overall health, and aromatherapy can be a valuable tool in supporting restful and restorative sleep. This section will delve into essential oils known for their sleep-promoting and relaxation benefits, such as lavender, cedarwood, and ylang-ylang. It will also guide you in creating a calming bedtime routine using essential oils, including diffuser blends and pillow sprays.
1. **Diffusion:** Using a diffuser in your bedroom can help create a calming environment conducive to restful sleep. Add sleep-promoting essential oils like lavender, cedarwood, or ylang-ylang to your diffuser and enjoy the soothing scents as you drift off to sleep.
2. **Topical Application:** Apply sleep-promoting essential oils diluted with carrier oil to your pulse points, such as wrists, temples, and behind your ears, before bedtime. It allows the relaxing scents to linger and help you unwind as you prepare for sleep. For example, blend a few drops of lavender essential oil with a carrier oil and try gently massaging it into your skin at pulse points to promote relaxation.
3. **Aromatherapy Bath:** Add sleep friendly essential oils like lavender, cedarwood, or ylang-ylang to your bathwater, along with Epsom salts or carrier oil, to create a soothing and relaxing bath experience before bedtime.
4. **Pillow Spray:** Combine a few drops of sleep friendly essential oils with distilled water in a spray bottle to create a calming pillow spray. Mist your pillow and bedding before sleep to help encourage relaxation and restful sleep. Lavender, cedarwood, and ylang-ylang essential oils work well for this purpose.

5. **Inhalation:** Inhaling sleep-promoting essential oils can help relax your mind and prepare your body for rest. Place a few drops of lavender, cedarwood, or ylang-ylang oil onto a tissue or cotton ball and inhale deeply. Add the oil to a personal inhaler or aromatherapy necklace for on-the-go relaxation.
6. **Bedtime Diffuser Blend:** Create a custom diffuser blend using sleep-promoting essential oils to help you unwind and prepare for a restful night's sleep. Combine lavender, cedarwood, and ylang-ylang essential oils in your diffuser and create an atmosphere for calm in your bedroom.
7. **Massage Oil:** Combine sleep friendly essential oil with carrier oils to create a relaxing massage oil. Gentle massaging with lavender, cedarwood, or ylang-ylang essential oils can help ease tension and promote relaxation before bedtime.

# Focus and Mental Clarity

Maintaining focus and mental clarity in a world of distractions can be challenging. Aromatherapy can help improve concentration and cognitive function by using specific essential oils. This section will discuss essential oils known for enhancing focus and mental clarity, such as rosemary, peppermint, and basil, and provide suggestions for incorporating these oils into your daily routine to support productivity and mental acuity.

1. **Diffusion:** Using a diffuser in your workspace or study area can help create an environment conducive to focus and mental clarity. Add focus-enhancing essential oils like rosemary, peppermint, or basil to your diffuser, and enjoy the stimulating scents as you work or study.
2. **Topical Application:** Apply focus-enhancing essential oils diluted with carrier oil to your pulse points, such as wrists, temples, and behind your ears, to help maintain concentration throughout the day. For example, mix a some drops of rosemary essential oil with a carrier oil and massage it into your skin to promote mental alertness.
3. **Aromatherapy Inhaler:** Create a personal inhaler using focus-enhancing essential oils to support mental clarity and concentration on the go. Blend a few drops of peppermint, rosemary, or basil essential oil and add the blend to a cotton wick in a personal inhaler, and inhale whenever you need a cognitive boost.
4. **Room Spray:** Enhance focus by combining few drops essential oils with distilled water in a bottle with a spray atomizer to create a refreshing room spray. Use this spray to refresh your workspace and encourage mental alertness.

5. **Focus-Boosting Blend:** Experiment with creating personalized essential oil blends that cater to your concentration and mental clarity needs. Combine focus-enhancing oils like rosemary, peppermint, and basil with uplifting oils like lemon or orange to create a balanced and mentally stimulating blend.

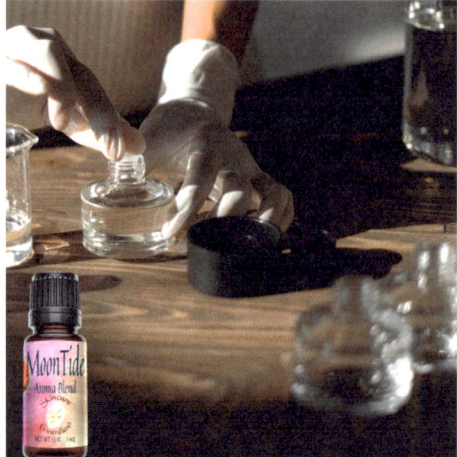

6. **Aromatherapy Jewelry:** Wear an aromatherapy necklace or bracelet to diffuse focus-enhancing essential oils throughout the day. Add a few drops of your favorite selections of essential oil to the jewelry's essential oil pad, and enjoy the stimulating aroma as you work or study.
7. **Massage Oil:** Combine focus-enhancing essential oils with carrier oil to create a stimulating massage oil. A gentle massage with rosemary, peppermint, or basil essential oils can help increase circulation and promote mental clarity.

# Personal Growth and Self-care

Embracing aromatherapy as a part of your self-care routine can be a powerful way to support personal growth and emotional well-being. By incorporating essential oils into mindfulness practices, meditation, and other self-care rituals, you can create a nurturing environment that fosters a deeper connection with yourself and your growth journey. In this section, we will discuss the importance of self-care and offer ideas for incorporating aromatherapy into your growing practices.

1. **Mindfulness Practices:** Mindfulness is being fully present and aware of the moment without judgment. Essential oils can help anchor your focus and create a soothing atmosphere for mindfulness exercises. Consider diffusing essential oils like lavender, frankincense, or bergamot during your mindfulness sessions to help promote relaxation and enhance concentration.
2. **Meditation:** Aromatherapy can enhance your meditation experience by stimulating the senses and creating a calming environment. Diffuse essential oils such as sandalwood, cedarwood, or patchouli to help ground you and deepen your meditation practice.

3. **Journaling:** Incorporating essential oils into your journaling routine can help evoke feelings of inspiration, clarity, and emotional release. Diffuse oils like rosemary, peppermint, or lemon stimulate creativity and clear the mind.
4. **Relaxation and Stress Relief:** Self-care is essential for maintaining balance and managing stress. Create a calming environment by diffusing essential oils like chamomile, ylang-ylang, or clary sage to promote relaxation and reduce feelings of stress or anxiety.
5. **Yoga and Exercise:** Aromatherapy can enhance your yoga or exercise routine by creating an uplifting and energizing atmosphere. Diffuse invigorating essential oils such as orange, eucalyptus, or grapefruit, to stimulate the senses and motivate you during your workout.

# Creating Personalized Essential Oil Blends

To support your unique emotional and spiritual needs, consider creating personalized essential oil blends that resonate with your growth journey. Begin by selecting a few essential oils that align with your goals, emotions, or desired state of mind. Experiment with various combinations and dilutions to find the perfect blend that meets your needs.

Some ideas for personalized blends include:

- **Emotional Balance:** Combine lavender, geranium, and frankincense to promote emotional stability and inner peace.
- **Confidence and Self-esteem:** Mix bergamot, jasmine, and rosemary to foster self-confidence and courage.
- **Focus and Clarity:** Combine rosemary, basil, and lemon to enhance mental clarity and concentration.
- **Spiritual Connection:** Mix frankincense, myrrh, and sandalwood to support spiritual growth and connection.

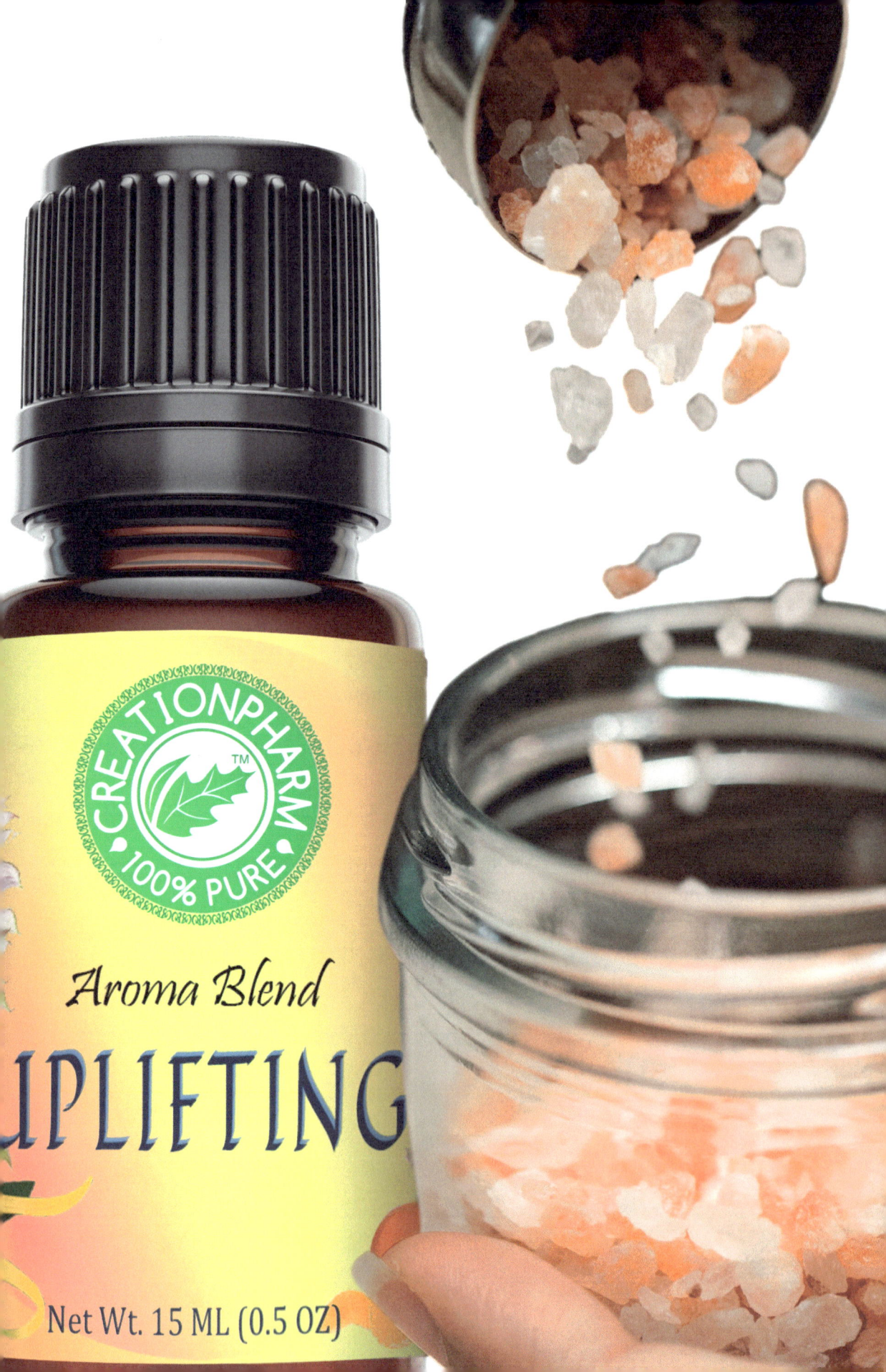

Chapter Eight

# Aromatherapy for Everyday Life

Aromatherapy is a versatile practice that can easily be incorporated into daily life. This section will explore various ways to use essential oils for everyday purposes, such as stress relief, relaxation, and focus. From diffusing essential oils in the home to adding them to skincare routines, aromatherapy can enhance physical, emotional, and mental well-being in various aspects of daily life.

## Creating a Morning and Evening Routine

Establishing a morning and evening routine with aromatherapy can set the tone for your day and help you unwind at night. This chapter will provide more in-depth guidance on creating personalized ways to support your goals and needs using essential oils.

**Morning Routine:** The morning is an ideal time to harness essential oils' uplifting and energizing properties. To begin your day with clarity and focus, consider incorporating the following steps into your morning routine:

**Morning Shower:** Before stepping in add a few drops of rosemary, eucalyptus, or peppermint essential oil to the shower floor. The steam will diffuse the oils, creating a refreshing atmosphere to help clear your mind and stimulate your senses.

**Diffuser Blend:** Use a diffuser to fill your living space with an energizing blend of essential oils. Citrus oils like lemon, grapefruit, and orange can promote a sense of alertness and boost your mood. Mixing these with rosemary or basil can enhance concentration and focus.

**Morning Meditation or Yoga:** Enhance your morning mindfulness practice by incorporating essential oils into your meditation or yoga routine. Try using frankincense or sandalwood for grounding or lavender and chamomile for relaxation.

**Evening Routine:** A soothing evening routine can help signal your body that it's time to unwind and prepare for restful sleep. Consider incorporating the following steps into your evening routine:

**Relaxing Bath:** Adding a few drops of chamomile, lavender, or ylang-ylang essential oil to your bathwater, along with a carrier oil like jojoba or MCT coconut oil. These calming oils can help ease tension and promote relaxation.

**Evening Diffuser Blend:** Create a calming environment by blending essential oils like lavender, cedarwood, and vetiver in your bedroom. These oils can help reduce stress, quiet the mind, and prepare your body for sleep.

**Bedtime Ritual:** Establish a bedtime ritual that includes the using essential oils. You can apply a relaxing blend to your temples, wrists, or the soles of your feet using a rollerball applicator. Alternatively, create a pillow spray with lavender, chamomile, or clary sage essential oils diluted in distilled water. Spritz your pillow and linens before bed to create a calming atmosphere.

# Aromatherapy in the Workplace

Aromatherapy can be a valuable tool in improving productivity, focus, and overall well-being in the workplace. This section will discuss the benefits of using essential oils at work, such as reducing stress, increasing concentration, and promoting a positive environment.

It will also guide you on incorporating essential oils into your workspace, including using personal diffusers, creating custom blends, and establishing aromatherapy-friendly policies.

## Aromatherapy in the Workplace

The workplace can often be a source of stress and mental fatigue. Integrating aromatherapy into your work environment can help enhance productivity, focus, and overall well-being. This section will delve deeper into the benefits of using essential oils at work and offer practical tips for incorporating them into your workspace.

## Benefits of Aromatherapy in the Workplace

Boost your workday with the power of essential oils. Use lavender, bergamot, and ylang-ylang to reduce stress and create a calm atmosphere. Enhance your concentration and focus with rosemary, peppermint, and lemon. Create a positive work environment with uplifting essential oils like grapefruit, orange, or jasmine.

## Incorporating Essential Oils into Your Workspace

1. **Personal diffusers**: These are an easy way to enjoy the benefits of dispersing essential oils in your work zone. Choose oils that support your work goals, such as improving focus, boosting creativity, or reducing stress.
2. **Custom Blends:** Create essential oil blends tailored to your needs. For example, you can mix lavender and rosemary to encourage relaxation and promote focus.

Store your combinations in small rollerball bottles for easy application throughout the day.
3. **Aromatherapy-Friendly Policies:** If you work in a shared office space or an open-plan environment, you must be mindful of your coworkers' preferences and sensitivities. Establish aromatherapy-friendly policies that include guidelines for appropriate essential oil use, such as using personal diffusers with a limited range or opting for less potent oils.

# Travel and On-the-Go Applications

Traveling can be both exciting and stressful. This section will explore how aromatherapy can support you during your travels, from easing motion sickness to promoting calm and relaxation during long flights. It will provide tips on packing essential oils for a trip, including how to safely transport your oils, and discuss various on-the-go applications, such as using inhalers, rollerballs, and portable diffusers to make the most of your aromatherapy experience.

## Travel and On-the-Go Applications

Travel can be a mix of excitement and stress, with factors like jet lag, motion sickness, and unfamiliar environments affecting your overall well-being. Aromatherapy can provide support during your journeys, helping you maintain balance and comfort. This section will discuss the benefits of using essential oils while traveling, offer tips for packing and transporting your oils, and explore various on-the-go applications to make the most of your aromatherapy experience.

## Benefits of Aromatherapy during Travel

- **Travel Comfortably**: Essential oils like ginger, peppermint, or spearmint can ease motion sickness during flights, car rides, or cruises.
- **Relax and Unwind**: Lavender, chamomile, and neroli can help promote calm and relaxation during travel.
- **Beat Jet Lag**: Essential oils like lavender, Roman chamomile, and vetiver can support sleep and help adjust to new time zones.
- **Stay Healthy**: Tea tree, eucalyptus, and lemon oils have antimicrobial properties that can boost your immune system while traveling.

# Packing and Transporting Essential Oils

- **Protect Your Oils**: Pack essential oils in a padded, protective case or wrap them individually to prevent breakage.
- **Avoid Leakage**: Use leak-proof bottles and ensure they are tightly sealed before packing.
- **Follow Regulations**: Check airline regulations for liquids in carry-on luggage, pack oils in containers that meet the size requirements, and place them in a clear, resealable plastic bag.

# On-the-Go Aromatherapy Applications

- **Inhalers**: Easy-to-use aromatherapy inhalers are perfect for travel. Load with your chosen essential oil and inhale as needed for benefits.
- **Rollerballs**: Apply essential oils topically without carrier oils with travel-friendly rollerball bottles. Customize blends for relaxation, motion sickness, or immune support.
- **Portable Diffusers**: Bring the benefits of aromatherapy on the go with battery-operated or USB-powered travel diffusers.
- **Wipes and Sprays**: Quick and easy aromatherapy on the go with essential oil-infused wipes and sprays. Use wipes to clean surfaces and sprays to refresh linens or as a facial mist.

# Aromatherapy for Special Occasions

Essential oils can take your special occasions, such as weddings, parties, and holidays, to the next level by creating a unique sensory experience that enhances the event's theme and ambiance. This section will provide ideas for integrating aromatherapy into your celebrations and guidance on selecting suitable essential oils to support the desired mood and atmosphere.

## Wedding

Make your wedding day unforgettable with aromatherapy! Enhance the atmosphere and create lasting memories for you and your guests by incorporating essential oils into your special day.

Choose from custom diffuser blends, scented party favors, and relaxation techniques using calming essential oils like lavender or bergamot. Create a signature scent for your wedding, offer essential oil-infused favors, and provide rollerball blends or small inhalers to promote a sense of calm during potentially stressful moments. Elevate the atmosphere and make your wedding even more memorable with the power of aromatherapy.

## Parties and Social Gatherings

Attention party hosts! Elevate your next gathering with the power of essential oils. Here are some creative ideas to incorporate aromatherapy into your event:
- Create a custom diffuser blend for the perfect ambiance.
- Add essential oils to invitations and/or decorations to enhance your theme.
- Set up an interactive DIY essential oil station for a fun party activity.
- Infuse cocktails, mocktails, and hand towels with refreshing or cozy essential oils.
- Incorporate essential oils into party games and icebreakers to engage guests.
- Thank your guests with gift bags filled with essential oil-infused goodies. Make your next gathering a memorable experience for everyone with the power of aromatherapy.

## Holidays

Enhance your holiday celebrations with aromatherapy! Create a festive atmosphere using holiday-themed diffuser blends or adding essential oils to decorations. Make personalized necessary oil gifts for loved ones. Get unique gift ideas and find calm during stressful times. Plus, check out eight more ways to incorporate essential oils into your holidays.
- **Aromatherapy Advent Calendar:** Discover new holiday scents each day with a unique advent calendar filled with essential oil samples.
- **Essential Oil Holiday Potpourri:** Create a customized holiday potpourri with dried fruits, spices, and essential oils for a festive touch.
- **Scented Holiday Baking:** Add a twist to traditional holiday treats with food-grade essential oils in your baking.
- **Aromatherapy Stocking Stuffers:** Surprise your loved ones with small essential oil items as stocking stuffers.
- **Essential Oil Room Sprays:** Freshen up your home with holiday-themed room sprays made with essential oil blends.
- **Aromatherapy Bath Salts:** Create luxurious and fragrant bath salts with Epsom salts, baking soda, and holiday essential oils.
- **Scented Gift Wrapping:** Infuse gift wrapping materials with essential oils for an extra sensory experience when opening presents.
- **Aromatherapy for Stress Relief:** Use calming essential oils like lavender or chamomile to reduce holiday stress and promote relaxation.

## Selecting Essential Oils for Your Special Occasion

Create the perfect atmosphere for your special occasion with essential oils. Consider these factors when choosing essential oils for your special occasion: desired mood and atmosphere, event theme, personal preferences and sensitivities, and seasonal considerations. Opt for gentle scents that cater to your guests' preferences and the occasion's music while also being mindful of potential sensitivities. Choose wisely for a memorable experience.

## Cultural and Regional Influences

Add cultural and regional scents to your special occasion for a unique sensory experience. For example, a Mediterranean-inspired event can feature olive, rosemary, or oregano essential oils. Careful selection can enhance the celebration and leave a lasting impression on guests, contributing to a successful event and creating a memorable atmosphere.

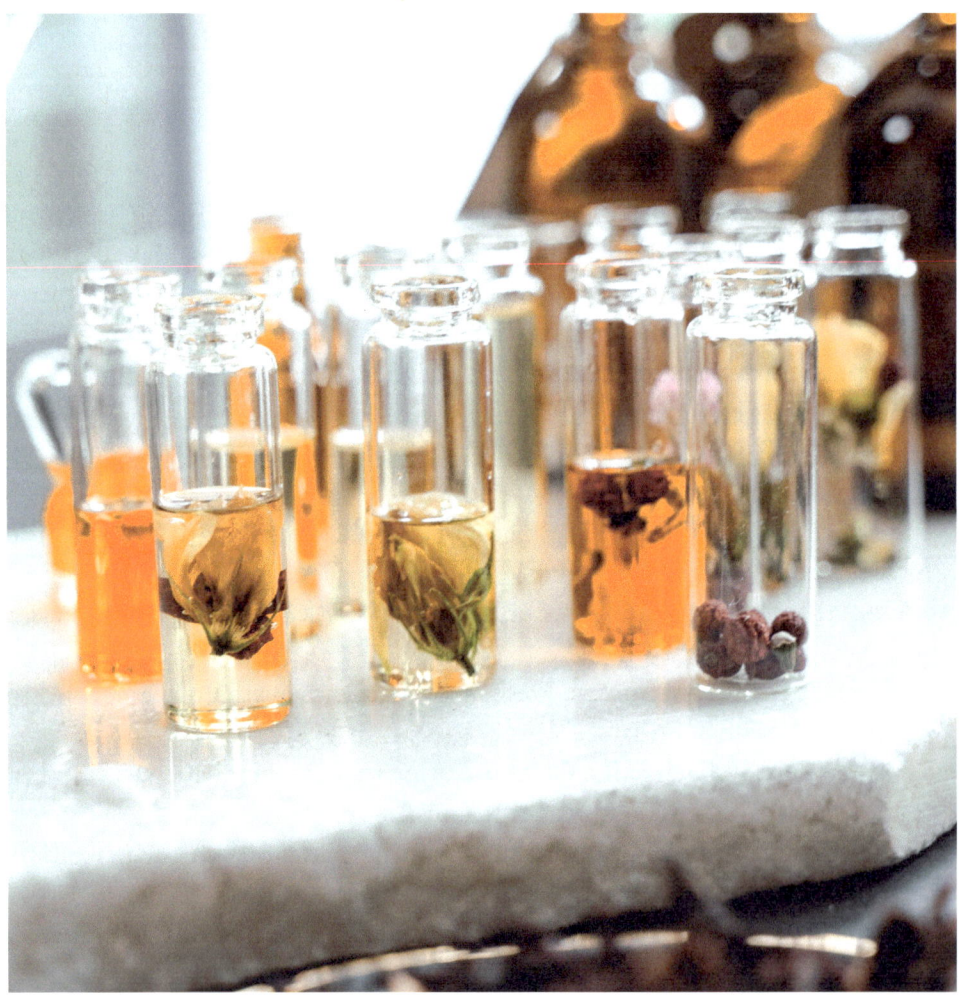

Chapter Nine

# Aromatherapy for Home and Environment

Discover the benefits of using aromatherapy to create a pleasant and healthy environment in your home. Essential oils offer a natural and effective alternative to harsh chemical cleaning products. This chapter will discuss various ways to use essential oils in your cleaning routine and provide recipes for creating your cleaning solutions.

## Natural Cleaning Solutions

Natural cleaning solutions are becoming increasingly popular as people seek healthier, more eco-friendly alternatives to traditional cleaning products. These solutions are made from natural ingredients such as vinegar, baking soda, and essential oils and effectively clean various home surfaces without harmful chemicals.

### All-purpose Cleaner

Create your all-purpose cleaner using water, a combination of antibacterial essential oils like lemon, tea tree, or eucalyptus, and white vinegar.

**Ingredients**:
• 1 cup water • 1 cup white vinegar • 15 drops lemon essential oil • 10 drops tea tree essential oil

**Instructions:**
1. In a spray bottle, combine white vinegar, and water.
2. Add the essential oils and shake well to blend.
3. Spray the mixture on the surfaces and wipe clean using a clean cloth.

### Surface Disinfectant

Learn to make using essential oils a natural spray with disinfectant and antimicrobial properties, such as lavender, thyme, or peppermint.

**Ingredients:**
• 1 cup water • ¼ cup rubbing alcohol or witch hazel • 8 drops each: lavender essential oil, thyme essential oil, and Tea Tree or Peppermint essential oil.

**Instructions:**
1. Combine water and rubbing alcohol or witch hazel in a spray bottle.
2. Add the essential oils and shake well to blend.
3. Spray the mixture on areas to clean and allow it to sit for a few minutes before wiping away with a clean cloth.

## Freshening laundry

Adding a few drops of your an appropriate essential oil or blend to wool dryer balls or a damp cloth can naturally add aroma your laundry and eliminate other smells.

**Ingredients:**
• Wool dryer balls or a damp cloth • Your choice of essential oil (e.g., lavender, lemon, or eucalyptus)

**Instructions:**
1. Try adding a few drops of essential oil to wool dryer balls or a damp cloth.
2. Toss the treated dryer balls or cloth into the dryer with your laundry load.
3. Enjoy the aroma after drying your laundry as usual.
Additional possibilities for natural cleaning solutions include:

## Glass and Mirror Cleaner

**Ingredients:**
• 2 cups water • 2 cups white vinegar • 15 drops peppermint essential oil

**Instructions:**
1. Combine water and white vinegar in a spray bottle.
2. Add the essential oil and shake well to blend.
3. Spray the mixture to clean glass surfaces and mirrors, wiping dry with a lint-free cloth.

## Carpet Deodorizer

**Ingredients:**
• 1 cup baking soda (sodium bicarbonate) • 25 drops of your favorite essential oil (e.g., lavender, lemon, or rosemary)

**Instructions:**

1. Combine essential oils and baking soda in a jar or vessel.
2. Blend/stir until the essential oil is evenly incorporated.
3. Sprinkle the mixture onto carpets, wait for 10-15 minutes.
4. Vacuum the carpet to remove the baking soda and leave behind a fresh aroma.

# Creating a Relaxing and Inviting Atmosphere

Essential oils can be used to create a calming and welcoming environment in your home. This section will provide ideas and guidance on:

- **Diffuser blends:** Discover how to create custom diffuser blends to suit the mood of each room in your home, such as energizing blends for the living room or calming blends for the bedroom.
- **Scented candles and potpourri:** Learn how to make your own scented candles or potpourri using essential oils to add a pleasant aroma to your living space.
- **Linen sprays and sachets:** Create your own linen sprays and sachets with essential oils to freshen up your bedding, closets, and drawers.

# Diffusing Essential Oils

Using an essential oil diffuser is a simple and effective way to create a pleasant atmosphere in your home. Diffusers release essential oils into the air, allowing you to enjoy their therapeutic benefits and create a welcoming environment. Choose calming and soothing oils like lavender, chamomile, or ylang-ylang for relaxation, or uplifting and invigorating oils like lemon, orange, or peppermint to energize your space.

**1. Cozy Winter Hearth Blend**
• 6 drops Orange • 2 drops Cinnamon • 2 drops Clove Leaf

**2. Refreshing Citrus Comforts**
• 4 drops Lemon • 3 drops Grapefruit • 4 drops Lime

**3. Calming Forests**
• 4 drops Pine • 4 drops Cedarwood • 3 drops Eucalyptus

**4. Exotica**
• 5 drops Ylang-Ylang • 4 drops Jasmine • 4 drops Sandalwood

**5. Flower Garden Bliss**
• 6 drops Lavender • 4 drops Geranium • 3 drops Roman Chamomile

**6. Sweet & Spicy**
• 6 drops Bergamot • 2 drops Cinnamon • 3 drops Vanilla

**7. Uplifting Springs**
• 4 drops Peppermint • 6 drops Lemon • 3 drops Rosemary

**8. Tranquility Gardens**
• 6 drops Lavender • 3 drops Clary Sage • 4 drops Bergamot

**9. Sensuality & Romance**
• 6 drops Patchouli • 4 drops Ylang-Ylang • 1 drops Rose

**10. Warmer and comfy**
• 6 drops Frankincense • 3 drops Myrrh • 2 drops Blood Orange

These essential oil blends can be added to your diffuser to create a warm and inviting atmosphere in your home. Adjust the number of drops to suit your personal preferences and the size of your space. Always follow the manufacturer's directions for your specific diffuser.

# Room Sprays

Create a custom room spray using water, witch hazel, and your favorite essential oils. This is an easy way to refresh the air and add a pleasant scent to your home. Simply combine 1 cup of water, ⅓ cup of witch hazel, and 18-36 drops of essential oils in a spray bottle, and shake well. Spray throughout your home to create an inviting atmosphere.

**1. Breezy Morning Air**
• 6 drops Lemon • 4 drops Eucalyptus • 4 drops Grapefruit • 4 drops Lavender

**2. Invigoration Retreat**
• 6 drops Rosemary • 3 drops Peppermint • 4 drops Basil • 4 drops Lime

**3. Serenity Sunset**
• 6 drops Lavender • 4 drops Orange • 6 drops Bergamot • 4 drops Geranium

### 4. Tropic Getaway
• 10 drops Virgin Coconut (warmed to liquefy) • 6 drops Lime • 6 drops Sweet Orange • 4 drops Ylang-Ylang

### 5. Magical Forest
• 6 drops Pine • 6 drops Cedarwood • 4 drops Cypress • 4 drops Juniper Berry

### 6. Spiced Citrus Delicata
• 6 drops Sweet Orange • 6 drops Lemon • 2 drops Cinnamon • 2 drops Clove bud oil

To make a homemade room spray using these essential oil blends, add the desired number of drops to a 4 oz (120 ml) glass spray bottle (with atomizer cap) and fill with distilled water. Add 1-2 tablespoons of witch hazel or alcohol to help the oils distribute in the water. Shake well before each use as the oils will separate from the water when it sits a while, and spray in your living space as desired to create an inviting atmosphere. Adjust the number of drops to suit your personal preferences and the size of your space.

## Scented Decor

Incorporate essential oils into your home decor by adding a few drops to potpourri, dried flower arrangements, or decorative pillows. This not only adds a subtle fragrance to your living space but also creates visual interest.

### 1. Vanilla Spicy Burn
• 6 drops Vanilla absolute (diluted) or Vanilla Extract • 3 drops Cinnamon • 6 drops Sweet Orange • 3 drops Clove

**Craft Idea:** Scented Pine Cone Decorations Collect pine cones and clean them. In a small bowl, mix the essential oils with 1 tablespoon of desired carrier oil (like sweet almond oil or jojoba). Brush the oil blend gently on the pine cones, and let them dry. Arrange the pine cones in a decorative bowl or basket creating a warm and inviting addition to your atmosphere.

### 2. Floral Forest Bliss
• 6 drops Lavender • 5 drops Geranium • 4 drops Jasmine • 4 drops Ylang-Ylang

**Craft Idea:** Scented Drawer Sachets Mix the essential oils with 2 cups of dried botanicals (like lavender, rose petals, or chamomile). Fill small simple fabric pouches with the scented mixture, and tie or sew them closed. Place the sachets in drawers, closets, or other areas to create a lovely, inviting scent.

### 3. Earthbound & Elegant
• 6 drops Sandalwood • 6 drops Patchouli • 4 drops Frankincense • 4 drops Vetiver

**Craft Idea:** Scented Wood Decor Purchase or gather small wooden pieces (such as branches, twigs, or driftwood). Mix the essential.

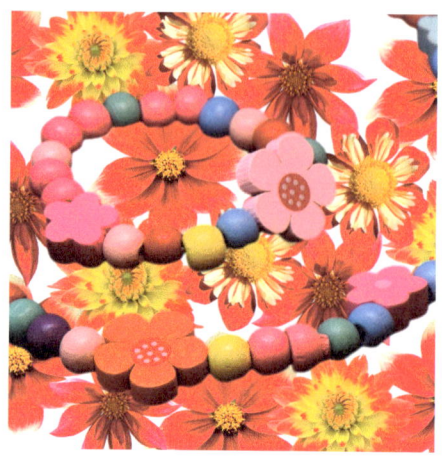

## Linen and Pillow Sprays

Create a calming bedtime atmosphere by using essential oils in linen and pillow sprays. Combine 1 cup of water, ⅓ cup of witch hazel, and 10-20 drops of lavender and/or chamomile essential oil in a spray bottle. Lightly mist your sheets and pillows before bed to encourage relaxation and restful sleep.

Creating pillow and linen sprays with essential oils is an easy and effective way to freshen up your home and promote relaxation. Here are four soothing aromatherapy blends that you can use to create your own linen and pillow sprays:

### 1. Lavender Night Blend
• 8 drops Lavender essential oil • 6 drops Chamomile essential oil • 4 drops Bergamot essential oil

### 2. Citrusly Uplifting
• 8 drops Sweet Orange essential oil • 8 drops Lemon essential oil • 4 drops Pink Grapefruit essential oil

### 3. Mint Refresher Blend
• 8 drops Peppermint essential oil • 6 drops Eucalyptus essential oil • 6 drops Rosemary essential oil

### 4. Wild Wilderness Blend
• 8 drops Cedarwood essential oil • 8 drops Sandalwood essential oil • 6 drops Frankincense essential oil

## Instructions for Making Pillow and Linen Sprays

**You will need:**
• A 4 oz (120 ml) dark glass spray bottle • Distilled water • 2 tablespoons witch hazel or vodka • Essential oil Blends (choose one of the above blends)

**Steps:**

1. In a small vessel, combine the witch hazel or vodka with the essential oil blend of your choice. Mix well to ensure they are mixed together.
2. Pour this mixture into the dark glass spray bottle.
3. Fill the spray bottle with distilled water, leaving a small gap at the top to prevent overflow.

## Aromatherapy Candles

Scented candles can add a warm and inviting glow to your home while also releasing the therapeutic benefits of essential oils. Look for candles made with natural soy or beeswax and scented with pure essential oils to ensure the best quality.

## Essential Oil Diffuser Jewelry

Incorporate essential oils into your daily life by using diffuser jewelry, such as necklaces or bracelets made with porous materials like lava stones or clay beads. Simply apply a few drops of your favorite essential oil or aromatherapy blend to the porous material on the jewelry away from any glaze or finish and enjoy the scent throughout the day.

Chapter Ten

# DIY Aromatherapy Recipes and Projects

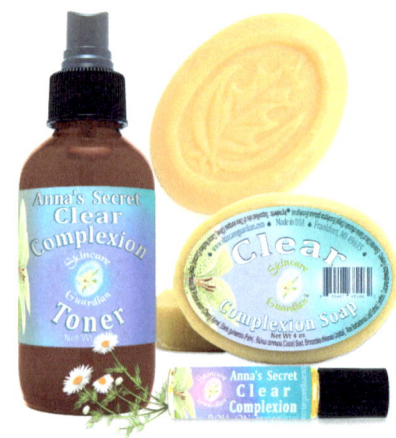

This chapter is devoted to providing readers with an array of recipes and projects that they can create using essential oils. Whether you are interested in creating personal care products, home fragrances, or gifts, this chapter has something for you. All the recipes and projects are easy to follow, and most of the ingredients can be found in your local natural food outlet or online.

## Personal Care Products

### Aromatherapy Massage Oil Ingredients

- ¼ cup carrier oil (like jojoba, or grapeseed oil)
- 8-15 drops of essential oil or aromatherapy blend of your choice

**Directions:**
1. In a small glass bottle, combine the carrier oil and essential oil.
2. Close the bottle and shake up a bit.
3. Store blends and massage oils in a cool, dark place.

Or consider these special blends:

### Universal Sports Massage Oil Ingredients

- 4 drops peppermint essential oil
- 4 drops eucalyptus essential oil
- 2 drops ginger essential oil
- ¼ cup jojoba

**Directions:**
1. Combine the essential oils and jojoba in a small glass bottle.

2. Close the bottle and shake up a bit to mix the oils.

3. To use, apply a small amount of the massage oil to the skin and massage into sore muscles.

## Study Hall Massage Oil Ingredients

- 6 drops rosemary essential oil
- 4 drops lemon essential oil
- 4 drops peppermint essential oil
- ⅓ cup sweet almond oil

**Directions:**
1. Combine the essential oils and almond oil in a small glass bottle.
2. Close the bottle and shake up a bit to blend the oils.
3. Apply a small amount of the massage oil to the skin and massage into your neck and shoulders to promote mental clarity and focus.

## Relaxer Massage Oil Ingredients

- 4 drops lavender essential oil
- 4 drops roman chamomile essential oil
- 4 drops bergamot essential oil
- ⅓ cup grapeseed oil

**Directions:**
1. Combine the essential oils and grapeseed oil in a small glass bottle.
2. Close the bottle and shake up a bit to blend the oils.
3. Apply a small amount of the massage oil to the skin and massage gently to promote relaxation and calmness.

## Stimulator Massage Oil Ingredients

- 4 drops black pepper essential oil
- 4 drops ginger essential oil
- 4 drops grapefruit essential oil
- ⅓ cup MCT coconut oil

**Directions:**
1. Combine the essential oils and MCT in a small glass bottle.
2. Close the bottle and shake up a bit to blend the oils.

3. Apply a small amount of the massage oil to the skin and massage gently to promote energy and alertness.

**Note:** When making massage oils, it's important to choose carrier oils that are easily absorbed. Jojoba oil, sweet almond oil, grapeseed oil, and MCT are great carrier oil options for massage oils. To make these massage oils, simply blend the essential oils with the carrier oil and mix well. Adjust the number of drops of essential oils to your liking, but be sure to follow safe dilution guidelines (usually 2-3% essential oil dilution for adults). Store the massage oils in a dark cool place and use within 4-6 months.

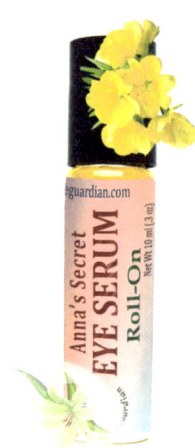

## Aromatherapy Bath Salts Ingredients

- 3 cups Epsom salt
- ½ cup baking soda
- 15-30 drops of essential oil of your choice

**Directions:**
1. In a suitable vessel for mixing, combine the Epsom salt and baking soda.
2. Add the essential oil and stir it up until blended well.
3. Storage in a glass jar with a tight-fitting lid is recommended.
4. To use, add ½ to 1 cup of bath salts to your bath and enjoy.

Or try one of these unique special bath salt recipes:

## Detox Bath Salts Ingredients

- 4 drops lemon essential oil
- 4 drops grapefruit essential oil
- 4 drops juniper berry essential oil
- 2 cups Epsom salt

**Directions:**
1. Combine the essential oils and Epsom salt in a large bowl to mix well and blend in the oils.
2. Add ½ to 1 cup of bath salts to your bathwater and soak for 20-30 minutes to promote detoxification and cleansing.

## Romantical Bath Salts Ingredients

- 4 drops ylang ylang essential oil
- 4 drops rose essential oil
- 4 drops sandalwood essential oil
- 2 cups sea salt

**Directions:**
1. Combine the essential oils and sea salt in a large bowl.
2. Blend the oils and salt together well.
3. Add ½ to 1 cup of bath salts to your bath and soak for 20-30 minutes for enhancement of relaxation and romance.

## Soothing Summer Bath Salts Ingredients

- 6 drops lavender essential oil
- 4 drops roman chamomile essential oil
- 6 drops frankincense essential oil
- 3 cups Himalayan pink salt (finely ground for easy dissolving)

**Directions:**
1. Combine the essential oils and Himalayan pink salt in a large bowl.
2. Blend well to mix in the oils.
3. Add ½ to 1 cup of bath salts to your bath and soak for 20-30 minutes to promote coolness, relaxation and calmness.

## Refreshing Bath Salts Ingredients

- 4 drops peppermint essential oil
- 4 drops rosemary essential oil
- 4 drops lemon essential oil
- 2 cups Dead Sea salt

**Directions:**
1. Combine the essential oils and Dead Sea salt in a large bowl.
2. Blend well to mix the oils.
3. Add ½ to 1 cup of bath salts to your bath and soak for 20-30 minutes to for a refreshing and energizing bath.

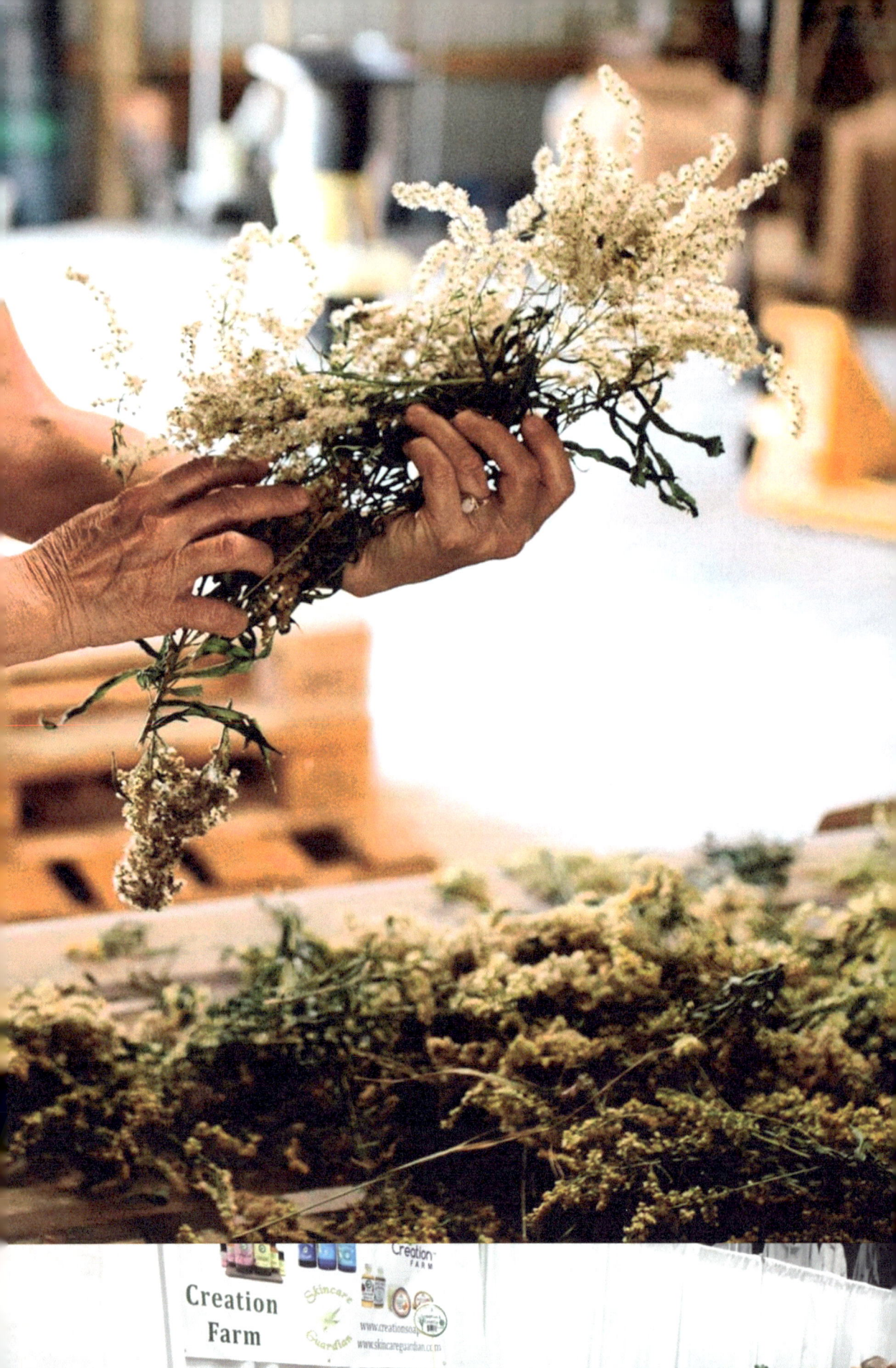

## Meditation Time Bath Salts Ingredients drops frankincense essential oil

- 6 drops cedarwood essential oil
- 4 drops myrrh essential oil
- 3 cups Epsom salt

**Directions:**
1. Combine the essential oils and Epsom salt in a large bowl.
2. Blend well to mix in the oils.
3. Add ½ to 1 cup of bath salts to your bathwater and soak for 20-30 minutes to promote meditation.

## Uplifting Bath Salts Ingredients

- 6 drops bergamot essential oil
- 6 drops orange essential oil
- 6 drops grapefruit essential oil
- 3 cups sea salt

**Directions:**
1. Combine the essential oils and sea salt in a large bowl.
2. Blend well to mix in the oils.
3. Add ½ to 1 cup of bath salts to your bath and soak for 20-30 minutes to promote uplifting spirits and energy.

**Note:** When making bath salts, it's important to choose salts that dissolve easily in water and are gentle on the skin. Epsom salt, sea salt, Himalayan pink salt, and Dead Sea salt are great salt options for bath salts. To make these bath salts, simply combine the desired essential oils to the desired salt and mix well. You can personalize abd adjust the number of drops of essential oils to your liking, but be sure to follow safe dilution guidelines (usually 2-3% essential oil dilution for adults).

## Ingredients for Aromatherapy Body Scrub

- 1 cup Epsom salt or Coarse sea salt
- ⅓ cup carrier oil (jojoba, or grapeseed oil)
- 8-15 drops of essential oil of your choice

**Directions:**
1. Combine the desired salt or and carrier oil in a small bowl.
2. blend the essential oil and salt and mix well.
3. Store in a glass jar with a tight-fitting lid.

4. Massage the scrub onto damp skin in a circular motion, then rinse off with warm water.

Here are some special body scrubs to try:

## Calmers Lavender Body Scrub Ingredients

- 6 drops lavender essential oil
- ⅔ cup sea salt
- ¼ cup Jojoba
- 1 tablespoon dried lavender flowers

**Directions:**
1. Combine the essential oil, sea salt, and Jojoba in a small bowl.
2. Blend well to mix in the oils and salt.
3. Add the dried lavender flowers and combine well.
4. Massage the body scrub onto damp skin in circular motions, eventually rinsing off with warm water.

## Energizer Citrus Body Scrub

- 6 drops lemon essential oil
- ⅔ cup sugar
- ¼ cup MCT
- ½ tablespoon grated lemon zest

**Directions:**
1. Combine the essential oil, sugar, and coconut oil in a small bowl.
2. Blend well to mix in the oils and sugar.
3. Add the grated lemon zest and combine well.
4. Massage the body scrub onto damp skin in circular motions eventually rinsing off with warm water.

## Refreshing Peppermint Body Scrub Ingredients

- 4 drops peppermint essential oil
- ⅔ cup Himalayan pink salt
- ¼ cup Extra virgin olive oil
- 1 tablespoon chopped fresh peppermint leaves

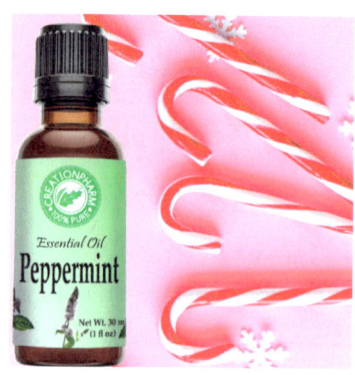

**Directions:**

1. Combine the essential oil, Himalayan pink salt, and olive oil in a small bowl.
2. Blend well to mix in the oils and salt.
3. Add the fresh peppermint leaves and mix well.
4. Massage the body scrub onto damp skin in circular motions eventually rinsing off with warm water.

## Rosemary Invigorating Body Scrub Ingredients

- 6 drops rosemary essential oil
- ⅔ cup brown sugar
- ¼ cup grapeseed oil
- 1 tablespoon chopped fresh rosemary leaves

**Directions:**

1. Combine the essential oil, brown sugar, and grapeseed oil in a small bowl.
2. Blend well to mix in the oils and sugar.
3. Add the fresh rosemary leaves and mix well.
4. Massage the body scrub onto damp skin in circular motions eventually rinsing off with warm water.

## Chamomile Soothing Body Scrub Ingredients

- 8 drops roman chamomile essential oil
- ⅔ cup oatmeal
- ⅓ cup jojoba
- 1 tablespoon dried chopped chamomile flowers

**Directions:**

1. Combine the essential oil, oatmeal, and jojoba oil in a small bowl.
2. Blend well to mix in the oils and oatmeal.
3. Add the dried chamomile flowers and mix well.
4. Massage the body scrub onto damp skin in circular motions eventually rinsing off with warm water.

## Grapefruit Exfoliator Body Scrub

- 8 drops grapefruit essential oil
- ⅔ cup coffee grounds
- ⅓ cup sweet almond oil
- 1 tablespoon grated grapefruit zest

**Directions:**

1. Combine the essential oil, coffee grounds, and almond oil in a small bowl.
2. Blend well to mix in the oils and coffee grounds.
3. Add the grated grapefruit zest and mix well.
4. Massage the body scrub onto damp skin in circular motions eventually rinsing off with warm water.

**Note:** When making body scrubs, it's important to choose ingredients that are gentle on the skin and provide effective exfoliation. Sea salt, sugar, Himalayan pink salt, and oatmeal are great exfoliants for body scrubs. Sweet almond oil, coconut oil, grapese

## Aromatherapy Hair Conditioner Ingredients

- ¼ cup apple cider vinegar
- ¼ cup distilled water
- 5-10 drops of essential oil of your choice

**Directions:**

1. Combine the apple cider vinegar and distilled water in a small bowl and mix well with the essential oil.
2. Transfer to a spray bottle.
3. After shampooing, spray the conditioner onto your hair and scalp and work in.
4. After treating with the rinse for a few minutes, rinsing off with warm water.

Below are three aromatherapy vinegar hair rinse recipes using various vinegars and herbs, and three essential oil blends in each:

## Lavender Cider Vinegar Hair Rinse Ingredients

- ½ cup apple cider vinegar
- ½ cup dried lavender flowers
- 6 drops lavender essential oil
- 3 cups water

**Directions:**

1. Bring the water to a boil in a small pan.
2. Removing from heat, add the cider vinegar and dried lavender flowers to steep.
3. Put a lid on the pan and let it steep for 25 minutes.
4. Strain the mixture through a fine-mesh strainer or filter into a clean jar.
5. Add the lavender essential oil and mix well.
6. After shampooing, pour the hair rinse onto your hair and scalp, massaging it in for a couple minutes, rinsing well with warm water.

## Rosemary White Vinegar Hair Rinse Ingredients

- ⅓ cup white vinegar
- ¼ cup fresh chopped rosemary leaves
- 6 drops rosemary essential oil
- 3 cups water

**Directions:**
1. Bring the water to a boil in a small pan.
2. Remove from heat and combine with the white vinegar and fresh rosemary leaves.
3. Put a lid on the pan and let it steep for 25 minutes.
4. Strain the mixture through a fine-mesh strainer or filter into a clean jar.
5. Add in the rosemary essential oil and blend well.
6. After shampooing, pour the hair rinse onto your hair and scalp, massaging it in for a few minutes, rinsing well with warm water.

## Peppermint Balsamic Hair Rinse Ingredients

- ⅓ cup balsamic vinegar
- ⅓ cup fresh peppermint leaves
- 6 drops peppermint essential oil
- 3 cups water

**Directions:**
1. Bring the water to a boil in a small pan.
2. Remove from heat, combine with the balsamic vinegar and fresh peppermint leaves.
3. Put a lid on the pan and let it steep for 25 minutes.
4. Strain the mixture through a fine-mesh strainer or filter into a clean jar.
5. Combine the peppermint essential oil and blend well.
6. After shampooing, pour the hair rinse onto your hair and scalp, massaging it in for a few minutes, rinsing well with warm water.

**Note:** When making Aromatherapy vinegar hair rinse, it's important to choose bemeficial ingredients that are beneficial for the scalp and hair. Apple cider vinegar, white vinegar, and balsamic vinegar, and rice vinegar are great options for hair rinses. Dried whole lavender flowers (mill in coffee mill) , fresh chopped rosemary leaves, and fresh chopped peppermint leaves are great herbs to use in hair rinses. To make hair rinses, bring the water and vinegar to a boil, add the herbs, and steep for 25 minutes. Filter the mixture and add the essential oils. Pour the hair rinse onto your hair and scalp after shampooing, massage it in, and rinsing well with warm water. Use the hair rinse once or twice a week.

## Aromatherapy Deodorant Ingredients

- ⅓ cup baking soda
- ⅓ cup cornstarch
- 10-15 drops of essential oil of your choice
- ⅓ cup coconut oil

**Directions:**
1. Combine the baking soda and cornstarch in a small bowl.
2. Mix in the essential oil and blend well.
3. Store in a glass jar with a tight-fitting lid.
4. Apply a small amount of the deodorant to your underarms to use.

## Falling Blossoms Deodorant Ingredients

- ⅓ cup baking soda
- ⅓ cup cornstarch
- 6 tablespoons coconut oil
- 12 drops lavender essential oil
- 12 drops geranium essential oil
- 12 drops ylang ylang essential oil

**Directions:**
1. Combine the baking soda and cornstarch in a small bowl.
2. Mix in the essential oil and blend well.
3. Store in a glass jar with a tight-fitting lid.
4. Apply a small amount of the deodorant to your underarms to use.

## Bursting Citrus Deodorant Ingredients

- ⅓ cup arrowroot powder
- ⅓ cup shea butter
- 6 tablespoons beeswax pellets
- 12 drops lemon essential oil
- 12 drops grapefruit essential oil
- 12 drops lime essential oil

**Directions:**
1. Melt the shea butter and beeswax pellets together in a double boiler.

2. Remove from heat and blend in the arrowroot powder, also combining the essential ois.

3. Move the mixture to a clean jar with a lid for storage.

4. Apply a pea-sized amount of deodorant to clean underarms to use.

## Goodsy Woods Deodorant Ingredients

- ⅓ cup baking soda
- ⅓ cup cornstarch
- 6 tablespoons cocoa butter
- 12 drops cedarwood essential oil
- 12 drops sandalwood essential oil
- 12 drops patchouli essential oil

**Directions:**

1. Mix the baking soda and cornstarch in a small bowl.
2. Add the cocoa butter and essential oils and stir until well combined.
3. Move the mixture to a clean jar with a lid for storage.
4. Apply a pea-sized amount of deodorant to clean underarms to use.

## Freshermint Deodorant Ingredients

- ⅓ cup arrowroot powder
- ⅓ cup coconut oil
- 6 tablespoons beeswax pellets
- 12 drops peppermint essential oil
- 12 drops eucalyptus essential oil
- 12 drops tea tree essential oil

**Directions:**

1. Melt the coconut oil and beeswax pellets together in a double boiler.
2. Remove from heat and blelnd in the arrowroot powder adding the essential oils and mixing well.
3. Move the mixture to a clean jar with a lid for storage.
4. Apply a pea-sized amount of deodorant to clean underarms.

**Note:** When making aromatherapy deodorants, it's important to choose ingredients that are gentle and safe on the skin and also help control body odor. Baking soda, cornstarch, and arrowroot powder are great options for absorbing moisture and controlling odor. Coconut oil, shea butter, cocoa butter, and beeswax are great options for diluting the essential ols,moisturizing the skin and holding the deodorant together. Lavender, geranium, ylang ylang, lemon, grapefruit, lime, cedarwood, sandalwood, patchouli, peppermint, eucalyptus, and tea tree are all efficient essential oils for deodorants. To make these deodorants, melt the ingredients together in a double boiler, remove from heat adding in the essential oils, and blending together well. Transfer the mixture to a clean jar with a lid and let it cool before using or putting on the lid for storage. Use by Applying a pea-sized amount of deodorant to clean underarms.

Chapter Eleven

# Building an Aromatherapy Toolkit

Aromatherapy can become essential to your daily routine with the right tools and equipment. This chapter will guide you through building your aromatherapy toolkit.

## Essential Oils and Carrier Oils

To begin with, you need a collection of essential and carrier oils that can be used for different purposes. Consider purchasing oils that are high-quality, pure, and organic. Here are some essential oils and carrier oils that can be included in your toolkit:

**Essential Oils:**
- Lavender
- Peppermint
- Eucalyptus
- Tea Tree
- Lemon
- Rosemary
- Geranium
- Ylang Ylang
- Chamomile
- Frankincense

**Carrier Oils:**
- Sweet almond oil is a popular carrier oil in aromatherapy and skincare.
- Jojoba oil resembles natural oils produced by the body for our skin and is excellent to balance oily skin.
- Grapeseed oil is light, non-greasy, and rich in antioxidants.
- Coconut oil has antibacterial and antifungal properties and can improve skin texture.
- Argan oil is luxurious and nourishing, great for dry and mature skin.
- Avocado oil is deeply moisturizing and can reduce inflammation and redness.
- Rosehip oil is high in vitamins, essential fatty acids, antioxidants, and is great for aging, dry, and/or damaged skin.

- Olive oil is rich in antioxidants, essential fatty acids and has antibacterial properties.
- Sunflower oil is easily absorbed, deeply moisturized, and has anti-inflammatory properties.

# Diffusers and Other Tools

Diffusers are an excellent way to enjoy aromatherapy in your home or workplace. Different types of diffusers are available, including ultrasonic diffusers, nebulizing diffusers, and reed diffusers. Choose a diffuser that suits your needs and preferences.

Other tools that can be useful in aromatherapy include:
- Aromatherapy jewelry
- Eye pillows
- Inhalers
- Roller bottles
- Spray bottles
- Mixing bowls and spoons

# Storage and Organization

For the longevity of your essential oils, storing them is necessary. Essential oils are highly concentrated distillate extractions that can be affected by environmental factors such as light, heat, and air exposure. Exposure to these factors can cause the oils to degrade and lose their potency over time, reducing their effectiveness in aromatherapy and skincare applications.

To store your essential oils properly, follow these tips:

1. **Store in a Cool, Dark Place**: Essential oils should always be stored in a cool, dark place away from direct sunlight and heat. The ideal temperature range for storing essential oils is 35-50 degrees Fahrenheit. You can store your essential oils in a cupboard, drawer, or refrigerator to keep them cool and protected from light.
2. **Use Dark Colored Glass Bottles**: Essential oils, such as amber or cobalt blue, should be stored in dark-colored glass bottles. These bottles help to protect the oils from very much light exposure which can cause the oils to degrade over time. Avoid storing essential oils in plastic bottles, as plastic can interact with the oils and alter their chemical composition.

3. **Keep the Caps Tightly Closed**: Essential oils should be stored with the caps tightly closed to prevent air exposure. Oxygen exposure can cause essential oils to oxidize, reducing their potency over time.
4. **Label Your Bottles**: It's important to label your essential oil bottles with the oil name, when you purchased, and any other pertinent information, such as variety of plant distilled or the source or quality range of the oil. This helps keep track of the oils and ensures you use the freshest oils possible.
5. **Keep Out of Reach of Children and Pets**: Keep essential oils out of reach of children and pets. Essential oils are highly concentrated and can be toxic if ingested. Always use caution when handling essential oils and store them in a secure location.

Essential oils can transform your daily routine into a self-care ritual, providing a sense of calm, balance, and rejuvenation. By incorporating aromatherapy into your everyday life, you can create a personalized experience that promotes physical, emotional, and spiritual wellness. However, it's important to remember that essential oils are highly concentrated plant distillations that require proper storage and handling to ensure their longevity and effectiveness.

While proper storage and organization may seem daunting, it's a simple and necessary step toward maintaining the quality and potency of your essential oils. By taking a few extra minutes to store your oils properly, you can ensure that they remain fresh and potent for longer, extending their shelf life and reducing waste.

Think of your essential oils as valuable treasures that deserve to be treated with care and respect. As you cultivate a collection of oils that resonate with you, it's necessary to store them in a way that honors their therapeutic benefits and ensures their longevity. Whether you are a seasoned aromatherapy enthusiast or just starting your journey, organizing and storing your essential oils can make a significant difference in the effectiveness and overall experience of using them.

So, embrace the art of organization and make it a part of your aromatherapy practice. With a little effort and intention, you can create a beautiful and functional space for your essential oils that inspire you to use them more often and appreciate their transformative power. Remember, a well-organized aromatherapy toolkit is not only practical but can also be a source of inspiration and motivation on your journey toward balance and wellness.

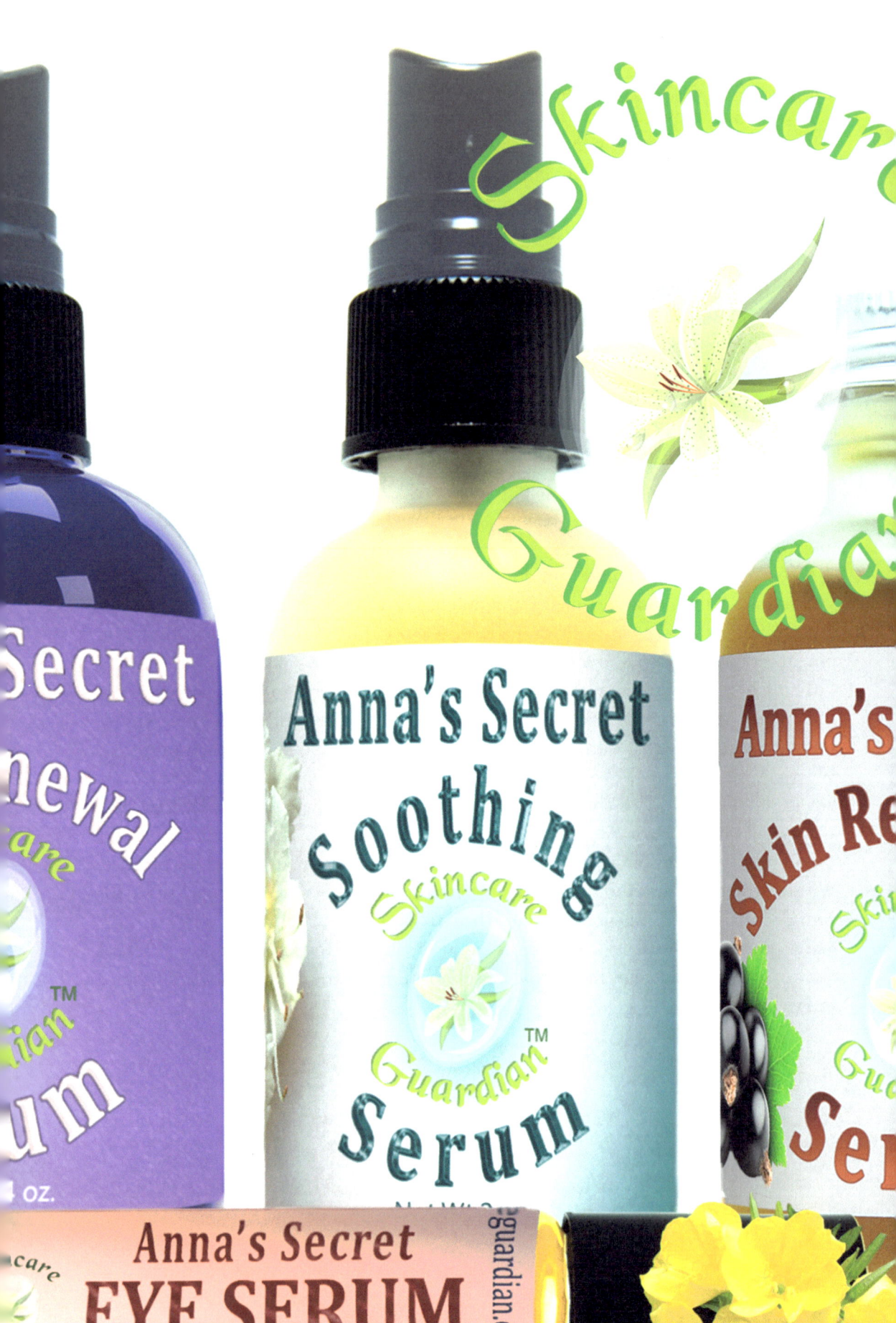

# Chapter Twelve

# The Future of Aromatherapy

Aromatherapy has a rich history that spans tens of centuries, yet its popularity continues to grow as people seek natural and holistic approaches to health and wellness. As the demand for essential oils and aromatherapy products increases, the future of aromatherapy looks bright, with exciting innovations and emerging research that support its effectiveness and potential.

Emerging research in aromatherapy is shedding light on the many therapeutic benefits of essential oils. Studies have shown that essential oils can be effective in reducing stress and anxiety, promoting relaxation and sleep, relieving pain and inflammation, improving cognitive function, and supporting immune function.

In addition to emerging research, there are also exciting innovations in the aromatherapy industry, such as new extraction methods that are more sustainable and efficient, as well as new delivery methods that offer unique and effective ways to experience aromatherapy. For example, essential oil diffusers have become increasingly popular in recent years, allowing people to enjoy the benefits of aromatherapy in their homes, offices, and other spaces.

Another area of innovation in aromatherapy is the use of technology to enhance the effectiveness of essential oils. For example, companies are exploring the use of micro-encapsulation to create essential oil products that release their scent slowly over time, providing longer-lasting aromatherapy benefits.

As the popularity of aromatherapy continues to grow, please consider the sustainability and ethical sourcing of our available essential oils. Sustainable and ethical sourcing practices not only protect the environment and the plants themselves, but also ensure the quality and potency of the oils. Many companies are committed to sustainable and ethical sourcing, working directly with farmers and distillers to ensure fair trade practices and environmental responsibility.

## Emerging Research and Innovations

Over the past few decades, research on the therapeutic benefits of essential oils and aromatherapy has increased, with promising findings that support their use in a variety of applications. Some of the emerging research includes:

**Antimicrobial Properties:** Essential oils have been found to have potent antimicrobial properties, with some oils showing efficacy against drug-resistant bacterial strains.
- **Anti-Inflammatory Effects:** Several essential oils have been shown to have anti-inflammatory effects, which may be useful in reducing inflammation in conditions such as arthritis and other chronic diseases.
- **Cognitive Function:** Certain essential oils have been found to have positive effects on cognitive function, such as improving memory and focus.
- **Pain Management:** Essential oils are believed to be effective in managing pain, with some oils showing promise in reducing the need for conventional pain medication.

In addition to emerging research, there are also exciting innovations in the aromatherapy industry, such as new extraction methods that are more sustainable and efficient, as well as new delivery methods that offer unique and effective ways to experience aromatherapy.

One area of emerging research in aromatherapy is its potential use in integrative medicine. Integrative and/or alternative medicine involves combining traditional medicine with complementary therapies, such as aromatherapy, to provide a more comprehensive approach to health and wellness. Aromatherapy is being explored as a complementary therapy in a variety of settings, including hospitals, clinics, and hospice care.

Studies have shown that aromatherapy can be effective in reducing pain and anxiety in hospital patients, improving sleep in cancer patients, and reducing symptoms of anxiety and depression in people with chronic conditions such as fibromyalgia and rheumatoid arthritis. Aromatherapy is also being explored as a potential treatment for conditions such as dementia and Alzheimer's disease.

In addition to its potential use in integrative medicine, aromatherapy is also being studied for its effects on mental health. For example, a study published in the Journal of Alternative and Complementary Medicine in recent years found that a blend of lavender, bergamot, and frankincense essential oils was effective in reducing symptoms of anxiety and depression in people with anxiety disorder.

As research in aromatherapy continues to emerge, it's also important to consider the wide potential of using essential oils to support health and wellness. However, it's also important to approach the use of aromatherapy with caution and to follow safe and responsible guidelines for use. Consulting with a healthcare professional or a certified aromatherapist can help ensure that you're using essential oils in a safe and effective way.

# The Growing Role of Aromatherapy in Integrative Medicine Aromatherapy

Aromatherapy is increasingly being recognized as a valuable new avenue of integrative and alternative medicine, which combines conventional medicine with complementary therapies to provide a comprehensive approach to health and wellness. Aromatherapy can be used in conjunction with other therapies such as massage, acupuncture, and chiropractic care to enhance their effectiveness and provide a more holistic approach to healing. Integrative medicine is a holistic approach to healthcare that focuses on treating the whole person, rather than just the symptoms of a specific condition. This approach involves combining traditional Western medicine with complementary and alternative therapies, including aromatherapy.

Aromatherapy has become an increasingly popular component of integrative medicine, as research has shown that it can be effective in treating a range of physical and mental health conditions. For example, studies have found that aromatherapy can be effective in reducing pain and inflammation, promoting relaxation and sleep, and improving cognitive function.

Aromatherapy is often used in combination with other complementary therapies, such as massage, acupuncture, and mindfulness practices, to create a comprehensive treatment plan for patients. This approach can be particularly beneficial for patients who are experiencing chronic pain, stress, or other chronic conditions that may not respond well to traditional medical treatments.

In addition to its therapeutic benefits, aromatherapy can also be a valuable tool for reducing medication use and improving patient outcomes. By incorporating aromatherapy into treatment plans, healthcare providers can potentially reduce the amount of medication needed to manage symptoms and improve patient satisfaction and quality of life.

As the role of aromatherapy in integrative medicine continues to grow, it's important for healthcare providers to be knowledgeable about the benefits and potential risks of essential oils, as well as proper usage and dilution guidelines. This can help ensure the safe and effective integration of aromatherapy into patient care plans.

# Aromatherapy and Sustainability

As the demand for essential oils grows, consider how sustainable they are and the need for ethical sourcing principles for these precious plant extracts. Sustainable and ethical sourcing practices not only protect the environment and the plants themselves but also ensure the quality and potency of the oils.

The increasing demand for essential oils and aromatherapy products has various effects on humanity, the world, economies, and cultures. One of the most significant impacts is on the environment, as the production and cultivation of essential oils can have both positive and negative effects.

On the positive side, the cultivation of plants for essential oil production can promote biodiversity and support local economies. Many essential oil plants are grown in developing countries, and the demand for these products can provide income for small-scale farmers and improve their livelihoods. Furthermore, sustainable cultivation practices can help preserve natural habitats and ecosystems, promoting the conservation of plant species and the protection of wildlife.

However, the demand for essential oils can also have negative effects on the environment if not managed sustainably. Over-harvesting, deforestation, and the use of harmful pesticides and chemicals can lead to the depletion of natural resources and damage to ecosystems. Additionally, the transportation of essential oils can contribute to carbon emissions and climate change.

Their is an essential need for sustainability in the production and sourcing of these precious oils and is therefore crucial for the future of essential oils. Companies will prosper who prioritize sustainability and ethical sourcing to help promote environmental responsibility and ensure the longevity of essential oil plants and their habitats.

The growing popularity of aromatherapy also has effects on economies and cultures. Aromatherapy and essential oils have become a booming industry, with many companies offering a wide range of products and services.

This industry provides jobs and income for many people, from farmers and distillers to retailers and therapists. Additionally, aromatherapy has become a part of many cultures, with traditions and practices around the use of essential oils and other natural remedies.

As the demand for natural and holistic approaches to health and wellness continues to grow, aromatherapy is likely to become even more integrated into cultures and economies around the world. However, it is essential to ensure that this growth is sustainable and responsible, both for the environment and for the people involved in its production and use.

Many companies are committed to sustainable and ethical sourcing, working directly with farmers and distillers to ensure fair trade practices and environmental responsibility. Additionally, some companies are exploring alternative sources of essential oils, such as plant-based synthetic options, which may provide a more sustainable and eco-friendly approach to aromatherapy.

The future of aromatherapy is bright, with emerging research and innovations that support its effectiveness and potential, as well as an increasing recognition of its role in integrative medicine and the importance of sustainable and ethical sourcing practices. As the popularity of aromatherapy continues to grow, it's important to stay informed and educated about the latest developments and to continue to use these precious plant extracts with respect, care, and intention.

The future of aromatherapy is indeed bright, as more and more people turn to natural and holistic approaches to health and wellness. The growing demand for essential oils has led to an increase in research and innovation, resulting in new and exciting discoveries about their therapeutic benefits and potential. As a result, the aromatherapy industry is constantly evolving, with new products, delivery methods, and extraction techniques being developed.

In addition to the many benefits of aromatherapy, there is also an increasing recognition of its role in integrative medicine. Many healthcare practitioners are now incorporating aromatherapy into their practices, recognizing its ability to complement traditional medical treatments and provide additional benefits to patients. This growing recognition of aromatherapy in healthcare is further supporting the growth and popularity of this practice.

However, as the demand for essential oils continues to grow, it's important to also consider the impact on the environment and the importance of sustainable and ethical sourcing practices. With many essential oils coming from rare or endangered plant species, it's crucial to ensure that they are sourced ethically and sustainably, to protect both the plants themselves and the ecosystems in which they grow.

Sustainable and ethical sourcing practices also ensure that the essential oils are of the highest quality and potency, providing maximum therapeutic benefits. By supporting sustainable and ethical sourcing, we are not only taking care of the earth but also supporting the livelihoods of farmers and distillers who depend on these plants for their income.

A BONUS FROM OUR SPONSOR

Scan code with your phone

# Conclusion

"Practical Aromatherapy for Everyday Living: A Comprehensive Guide to Essential Oils and Their Applications for a Balanced Lifestyle" is an essential resource for anyone interested in incorporating aromatherapy into their daily routine. This guide provides a comprehensive overview of essential oils, their therapeutic properties, and practical tips and techniques for using them safely and effectively.

One of the key takeaways from this guide is the importance of choosing high-quality, pure essential oils. By sourcing oils from reputable suppliers and using them correctly, readers can experience the full benefits of aromatherapy, including stress relief, improved mood, and enhanced physical well-being.

The guide includes various recipes and blends for different purposes, such as promoting relaxation, boosting energy, and improving focus and concentration. From diffusing oils in a bedroom to using them in massage or skin care, there are endless ways to incorporate aromatherapy into daily life.

"Practical Aromatherapy for Everyday Living" is a valuable resource for anyone looking to improve their well-being and create a more balanced, harmonious lifestyle. Whether you are a beginner or an experienced aromatherapy practitioner, this guide offers something for everyone and will become a go-to reference for years.

By learning about the power of essential oils, you can transform your daily routine and achieve greater physical, mental, and emotional well-being.

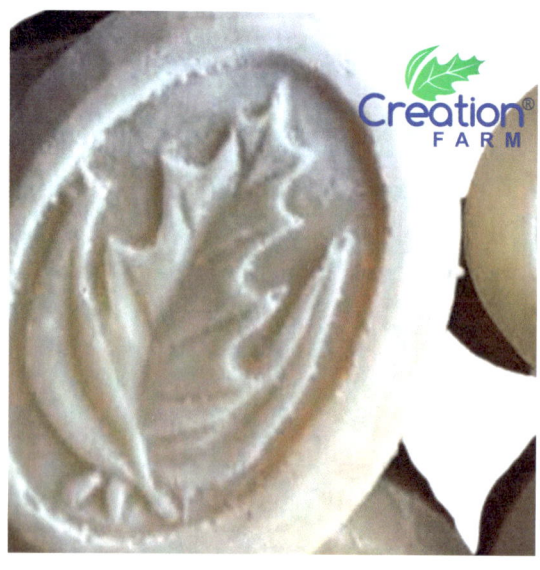

Made in the USA
Columbia, SC
01 October 2024